The
Activities
Catalog

A complete discussion of *The Activities Catalog* is available in a companion volume, **A Comprehensive Guide to *The Activities Catalog: An Alternative Curriculum for Youth and Adults with Severe Disabilities*.** This book comes packaged with one copy of *The Activities Catalog.* (Additional catalogs are available in packages of three.) To order the book or the catalogs, contact Brookes Publishing Co., P.O. Box 10624, Baltimore, MD 21285-0624.

The Activities Catalog

An Alternative Curriculum for Youth and Adults with Severe Disabilities

by

Barbara Wilcox, Ph.D.
and G. Thomas Bellamy, Ph.D.

Specialized Training Program
University of Oregon
Eugene

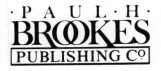
·P·A·U·L·H·
BROOKES
PUBLISHING CO

Baltimore • London

Paul H. Brookes Publishing Co.
P.O. Box 10624
Baltimore, Maryland 21285-0624

Typeset by Brushwood Graphics Inc., Baltimore, Maryland.
Manufactured in the United States of America by
Pavsner Press, Baltimore, Maryland.

Activities illustrations by Mark E. Danielson.

Cover design conceptualization contributed by Arden Munkres.

Library of Congress Cataloging-in-Publication Data
Wilcox, Barbara, 1947–
  The activities catalog.

  Includes index.
  1. Handicapped—Life skills guides. 2. Handicapped—
Recreation. 3. Handicapped youth—Life skills guides. 4. Handi-
capped youth—Recreation. I. Bellamy, G. Thomas. II. Title.
HV1568.W55 1987   646.7   86-29883
ISBN 0-933716-75-3

Introduction

Leisure

Personal Management

Work

Introduction

Ordering From the Catalog

These days, nothing in our mailbox is more common than a catalog. What's so unusual about this one?

The Activities Catalog is essentially a catalog of life's activities. No emotions, thoughts, or feelings, but the day-to-day events that keep us busy, healthy, and happy. *The Activities Catalog* displays: 1) the myriad of ways we might constructively use free time, 2) all those things that we might do to care for ourselves and contribute to our household, and 3) the various kinds of work we might do to earn wages and contribute to the community. In short, it is a catalog with three sections: leisure, personal management, and work.

The Activities Catalog is an alternate curriculum system for youth and adults with severe handicaps. It replaces traditional curriculum materials that emphasize isolated developmental or academic skills. *The Activities Catalog* emphasizes, instead, the stuff of adult life. Unlike most curricula, the catalog does not present a sequence of material to be taught and mastered. Basic to the catalog is the assumption that since we simply can't learn everything, decisions about what to teach an individual with severe handicaps are more dependent on values—of family, friends, advocates, and of course, the individual him or herself—than upon any logical sequence. *The Activities Catalog* acknowledges that choosing curriculum goals for an individualized plan poses the same dilemma as placing an order from a commercial catalog: there are many items that look desirable . . . but not enough resources to purchase everything.

The Activities Catalog is used, quite literally, to place an order of valued activities for an individual with a severe handicap. Review activities in each domain, decide which activities would increase his or her quality of life, fill out an order form, and turn it in at the individualized education program (IEP) or individual habilitation plan (IHP) meeting. As you place your order, strive to create a balanced life-style for your son, daughter, friend, student, worker, or housemate with a disability. Naturally, it is important to have some activity in each major domain. Also, since the categories that organize entries within each domain each represent activity groups that are important to a balanced life-style, you may want to order activities from each category.

Good luck! Decisions are always difficult. You'll find order forms at the end of the catalog, on pages 85, 87, 89, and 91.

The Activities

Each entry in the catalog contains a broad analysis that gives you an idea of the general components of the activity. If you see steps that seem very difficult or that you think your son or daughter (or student, or worker, or resident) will find troublesome, that does not mean the activity is impossible. It simply means one might have to modify the activity a bit, design some sort of prosthetic device or alternate performance strategy to compensate for the difficulty, or do some concentrated training on that particular activity step. The activity analysis also serves to help teachers or other training staff develop data sheets to monitor progress, and provides a framework for building instructional programs.

The activity analysis is intentionally broad. It is designed to be generic; that is, to describe the activity *anywhere* it occurs. Each component in the analysis represents a fairly large chunk of behavior. While these chunks can, of course, be broken down into smaller steps to fit specific people with disabilities or to fit particular settings, it would not make much sense for that to be done in the catalog itself.

Activities have a beginning, an execution, and an ending. Getting started and continuing on to something else once you're done is just as important as doing the activity itself. Each activity analysis includes components that emphasize that starting out and finishing up are important for individuals with severe handicaps as well!

In addition to the generic analysis, each activity entry also includes basic information on cost, equipment required, and common adaptations to make participation possible even though an individual might lack basic skills.

When one activity might be combined easily and appropriately with another, that is often noted as well.

Local Information

Naturally, when you order an activity from *The Activities Catalog* for an individualized education program or an individual habilitation plan, you will need to know when and where in your own community that activity is available. Unfortunately, the catalog cannot supply that information for you. You are on your own—but not entirely, of course. For details of activities in your community, consult the Yellow Pages, newspapers, brochures, advertisements, and, of course, your friends.

Using *The Activities Catalog* System

If you are interested in the background and rationale for *The Activities Catalog* and in how the catalog system meets other important curriculum functions such as assessment, the designing of intervention strategies, and program evaluation see *A Comprehensive Guide to The Activities Catalog: An Alternative Curriculum for Youth and Adults with Severe Disabilities.* (Wilcox & Bellamy, 1987). That companion volume has chapters that describe the application of *The Activities Catalog* in high schools, supported employment, and residential services for people with severe handicaps. It is available from Paul H. Brookes Publishing Company, P.O. Box 10624, Baltimore, MD 21285-0624 (Toll-free order number: 1-800-638-3775).

Suggestions?

If you have comments on *The Activities Catalog* we'd love to hear from you. Send them to:
Barbara Wilcox and Thomas Bellamy
c/o Paul H. Brookes Publishing Company
P.O. Box 10624
Baltimore, MD 21285-0624

Leisure

Exercise

See the community . . . and be seen!

Walking is an ideal way of introducing structure and exercise . . . without pain or equipment. Walking can be done at any time for virtually any length of time. It is an opportunity to be alone or to spend time with friends. Walking with a partner is a natural way to guarantee support necessary for crossing streets and dealing with unexpected events.

Activity includes:
- Selecting apparel appropriate for weather
- Traveling to destination/traveling for duration
- Returning to origin
- Continuing to next activity

Using Heavy Hands or spats can increase the workout!

A sequence of pictures identifying major landmarks or decision points on the route can promote independence while at the same time providing unobtrusive supports.

ITEM 1-1-1   Walking

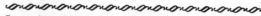

Restore human legs as a means of travel. Pedestrians rely on food for fuel and need no special parking facilities.
Lewis Mumford

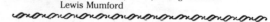

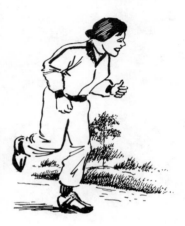

Minimum equipment. Maximum conditioning.

Jogging offers great flexibility. It can be done alone or with a group. It can be done virtually anywhere at any time.

Equipment requirements for this activity are minimal: well-fitting shoes, shorts, and top. Rain gear or outer clothing will be necessary for outdoor jogging at some time of year. A stopwatch is optional.

Activity includes:
- Selecting time and location for run
- Changing into appropriate clothing
- Doing stretching/warm-up exercises
- Jogging
- Showering
- Changing clothes
- Continuing to next activity

Running with a partner is a normal and unobtrusive way of providing support for participants. Organized "fun runs" offer individuals the opportunity to participate in a community-wide event, and provide the intermediate goals necessary to keep up the habit. Since registrants for fun runs usually get a t-shirt as well, jogging can contribute to the wardrobe!

Individual programs may focus on increasing speed or distance. Jogging is an ideal component of any weight reduction or conditioning effort.

ITEM 1-1-2   Jogging

Relaxation and transportation.

Bike riding is a way to keep fit and see the community. It can be done alone or with a group of friends.

Activity includes:
- Getting necessary materials (pant guard, reflectors, lock and key)
- Getting bike from storage
- Mounting and riding bike
- Returning to origin
- Returning bike and equipment to storage
- Continuing to next activity

Be sure to define where the individual will ride. There should be specific training to ensure that folks can respond to traffic and safety conditions that arise along target routes.

Bike riding for transportation will require an individual to use a lock and key to secure the bike at the destination. Training may also include bike maintenance or repair.

A three-wheeled bike adds stability for riders who lack balance, and is both functional and dignified.

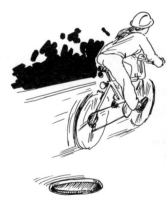

ITEM 1-1-3   Riding a Bike
    a. Exercise only
    b. Means of transportation

Take advantage of that lazy afternoon in the park— play catch with a ball or frisbee.

Activity includes:
- Getting ball/frisbee
- Inviting others to play
- Traveling to suitable playing area
- Tossing ball/frisbee
- Traveling home/to next activity
- Returning ball/frisbee to storage

Equipment is minimal, readily available, and inexpensive. The rules, length of the game, and number of participants are flexible. Easily accommodates players of all skill levels.

ITEM 1-1-4   Playing Catch

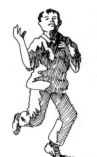

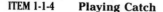

Learn skills that support health and fitness: Take a class!

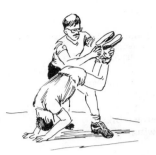

Depending on your community, class options may be endless. Two things will be typical: fees will be charged and specialized attire required.

While the routine will vary somewhat from class to class, in general this activity includes:

- Gathering necessary clothing/equipment
- Traveling to class
- Changing clothing
- Completing warm-up exercises
- Following instructor directives
- Changing clothes
- Traveling to next activity

To locate classes near you, check in the Yellow Pages, and park and recreation and community center bulletins. Classes typically meet once or twice per week.

Enrolling in a formal class is an ideal way to meet new friends in the community or maintain contact with old friends. Recruiting a "buddy" at the outset is a good way to ensure a successful class experience.

ITEM 1-1-5　Attending Skill-Building Classes
    a.　Gymnastics
    b.　Martial arts
    c.　Yoga

Note: This can be combined with ITEM 2-1-1: Using Restrooms.

Exercise. Therapy. Fun. All rolled into one!

Thanks to modern technology, you can swim year 'round in almost any climate.

Activity includes:
- Gathering swimsuit/swim trunks and other materials (towel, cap, goggles, nose clip, etc.)
- Traveling to pool
- Showing ID/pass or paying fee
- Finding locker/getting basket
- Changing into suit/trunks
- Storing clothing and other possessions
- Swimming
- Showering
- Dressing
- Collecting possessions/returning materials
- Traveling to next activity

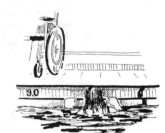

The equipment requirements for this activity are minimal: swimsuit/swim trunks (and perhaps a cap depending on individual pool requirements). Some pools provide suits/trunks and/or towels, so you may want to check before you go.

Most pools charge a fee. You may be able to purchase individual swims, a set of lessons or visits, or a season/annual pass.

The pool schedule will be a major factor in performing this activity, so be sure to get a copy of pool hours and a notice of any time or use restrictions (e.g., lap swimming only, women only).

Swimming offers opportunities for fun and individuals of all ability levels.

ITEM 1-1-6　Swimming
    a.　Lessons
    b.　Recreational

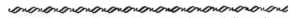
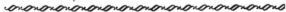

Increased means and increased leisure are the two civilizers of man.
Anonymous

Aerobic exercise classes are one of the fastest growing ways of keeping fit.

Aerobics classes are widely available both in high school physical education programs and at a variety of locations throughout a community. Morning, daytime, and evening sessions are available.

Participation may require payment of registration fees, transportation to the site, exercise clothing (warm-up suit or leotard or tights), sport shoes, a bag for transporting gear, and lock and key.

Activity includes:
- Preparing to go (getting bus pass, arranging transportation, etc.)
- Traveling to class
- Changing clothes
- Attending class and following routines
- Changing clothes
- Traveling to next activity

A common adaptation is to dress at home for a class at a community location. Both the instructor and other class members provide continuous modeling.

Individuals are urged to participate at their own level until they can keep up with the full routine. Classes typically accommodate individuals at different levels of fitness.

ITEM 1-1-7　Participating in Aerobics/Slimnastics/ Jazzercise Class
    a.　At school
    b.　At a community location

Note: This activity may include ITEM 2-1-1: Using Restrooms; and may be combined with ITEM 2-1-4: Dressing.

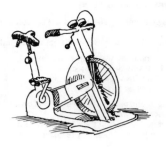

School. Home. Gym. There are many places where you can keep in shape (or get in shape) using exercise equipment.

This activity is limited only by the equipment available.

Activity includes:
- Changing into appropriate clothing
- Getting equipment from storage
- Using equipment
- Returning material to storage
- Showering and changing clothes as necessary
- Continuing to next activity

Users will need minimum instruction specific to each type of equipment. Consider programs to increase length of exercise period.

ITEM 1-1-8   **Using Exercise Equipment**
    a. **Jump-rope**   c. **Exercise bike**
    b. **Rebounder**   d. **Rowing machine**

Physical fitness is a must for the 80s . . . and weight training is an increasingly popular way to keep fit.

This activity can be done alone or with a small group of friends. Providing assistance and encouragement to one another is an integral part of the activity.

Activity includes:
- Traveling to weight-training area
- Changing clothes
- Adjusting weights/machines
- Working out with weights/machines
- Showering
- Changing clothes
- Continuing to next activity

Membership dues or fees may be required at community locations.
A sequence of photographs can prompt correct positioning and use of machines, as well as specify an optimal order for exercises to be completed.

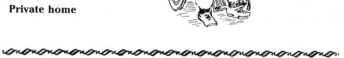

ITEM 1-1-9   **Weight Training**
    a. **High school physical education class**
    b. **Community recreation center or fitness club**
    c. **Private home**

When I was forty, my doctor advised me that a man in his forties shouldn't play tennis. I heeded his advice carefully and could hardly wait until I reached fifty to start again.
                  Justice Hugo Black

Tennis, anyone?

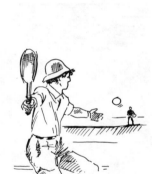

A variety of racquet sports offer opportunities for individual or team competition . . . or simply good fun.

Each of these activities requires some specialized equipment: racquet, shoes, ball/birdie, and a special playing area. Racquet sports are good leisure options when playing areas are easily available or when others in the family or neighborhood have an active interest in the sport.

Activity includes:
- Identifying a partner
- Gathering necessary materials
- Travel to playing area
- Playing/volleying
- Returning to origin
- Returning material/equipment to storage
- Continuing to next activity

While most racquet sports require two players, tennis and racquetball can be practiced individually against a backboard.

ITEM 1-1-10   **Playing Racquet Sports**
    a. **Tennis**   c. **Ping pong**
    b. **Racquetball**   d. **Badminton**

Different Reasons . . . Different Goals

There are several reasons that you might want to include an activity on a person's IEP or IHP. Very often we choose activities because they are things we would like the person to learn. We call those *acquisition* goals.

Sometimes, though, we include activities that an individual can already do because we want to change some aspect of his or her performance. Those *performance* goals might focus on ensuring opportunities to participate or on changing the quality of the performance. Examples of quality change goals might include training or support to make performance more integrated, intervention to increase the frequency of an activity or to increase the variety of circumstances under which the activity could be done, training for choice over certain activity components, or training to make performance more independent.

In *The Activities Catalog* system, goals related to the performance of valued activities are considered just as important as goals that target new learning.

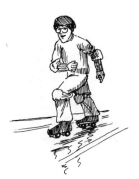

Skate the great outdoors . . . or your local rink.

Participation requires skates and a smooth surface. Most rinks rent skates for a small fee. Knee pads are nice, especially for beginners.

Activity includes:
- Preparing to go (checking appearance; getting skates, knee pads, money)
- Traveling to rink
- Paying fees (and renting equipment if necessary)
- Putting on skates
- Skating
- Changing to street shoes
- Returning rental equipment (if necessary)
- Returning to next activity

While constraints disappear if you elect to skate outside a formal rink, the social benefits may also be reduced.

Partners are a nice way to increase social integration and provide physical support.

ITEM 1-1-11 **Skating**
 a. **Roller skating**
 b. **Ice skating**

Note: This activity may incorporate ITEM 2-1-1: Using Restrooms and ITEM 2-2-4: Using Vending Machines.

The Same Activity Can Mean Many Things

The Activities Catalog simply presents activities. It's up to you to decide what they mean for the individuals you care about.

The same activity can have different implications for the life-style of different people. For example, "Using a Sit-Down Restaurant" might represent an opportunity for one individual to share an evening with an intimate friend. For another person, being able to eat out at a restaurant might be important in surviving in a household where a parent is not always home to prepare dinner.

Similarly, "Attending An Aerobics Class" might represent an important element in an individual health and fitness program or simply a pleasant activity to do with a friend on a Thursday night.

Consider each activity carefully. Think what it might mean to the person in question.

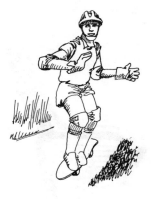

Thrills . . . and spills.
The skateboard has become part of the "teen scene," especially in milder climates.

Activity includes:
- Gathering necessary equipment (board and safety gear)
- Traveling to appropriate location
- Skateboarding
- Traveling home
- Returning equipment to storage
- Continuing to next activity

Though the sport looks simple enough, there are significant equipment requirements. Cost for the board itself can range from $20 to $70.

Just as important is the safety gear: elbow and knee pads are a must, and a helmet is strongly recommended.

This activity requires fairly good balance. An area with a smooth, flat surface is necessary for initial training.

Sidewalk etiquette and traffic rules are important once one leaves a designated training area.

ITEM 1-1-12 **Skateboarding**

To dance . . .

Well, why not! Dancing may not be for everyone, but it might be for you.
Dance classes are an excellent way to get and stay fit, and to broaden your circle of friends.

Activity includes:
- Putting on appropriate clothing
- Traveling to class
- Changing into appropriate footwear as necessary
- Dancing
- Changing back into street shoes if necessary
- Traveling to next activity

Classes are available through schools, continuing education programs, community centers, and private instructors. The fees, length, and schedule of classes will vary. Requirements for specialized clothing and shoes will depend on the type of class selected and the preference of the instructor.

ITEM 1-1-13 **Participating in Dance Classes**
 a. **Ballet** d. **Ballroom dancing**
 b. **Tap** e. **Folk dancing**
 c. **Jazz** f. **Square dancing**

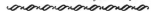

Those who decide to use leisure as a means of mental development, who love good music, good books, good pictures, good plays, good company, good conversation— what are they? They are the happiest people in the world.
William Lyon Phelps

11

Team sports are part of growing up.

There is great variety . . . and some of us have to be chosen last.

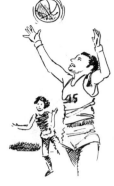

Activity includes:
- Dressing in appropriate clothing
- Gathering necessary equipment
- Traveling to playing field
- Playing
- Collecting equipment
- Traveling home/to next activity

May require additional time for practices and/or individual skill development activities. Most games require reasonable stamina, coordination, and speed, and involve some degree (more or less violent!) of physical contact.

Clothing, shoes, and equipment needs will depend on the sports selected. Schools, park and recreation programs, and community sports programs offer a range of opportunities.

ITEM 1-1-14   Playing Team Sports
a.	**Baseball/softball**	d. **Basketball**
b.	**Football/flag football**	e. **Volleyball**
c.	**Soccer**	

For the rest of us who like team sports—but not enough to risk physical damage—there's a perfect solution: Be a manager.

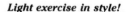

Every team needs someone to be responsible for equipment and supplies. Why not serve this important function at games or practices?

Activity includes:
- Gathering all necessary equipment
- Traveling to playing area
- Distributing equipment, towels, etc. as necessary throughout game/practice
- Collecting equipment
- Traveling back to point of origin
- Returning equipment to storage/laundry

A self-management checklist is an ideal aid for managing what may be a relatively complex task.

Contact individual team coaches or sports program offices to volunteer your services!

ITEM 1-1-15   Being a Team Manager

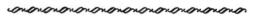

If you watch a game, it's fun. If you play it, it's recreation. If you work at it, it's golf.
Bob Hope

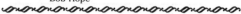

Light exercise in style!

Golf may not be the best way to work up a sweat but it is hardly a bad way to spend a weekday evening or weekend day—providing the weather cooperates. And, goodness knows, not everyone who plays comes close to playing well!

Activity includes:
- Dressing in appropriate clothing
- Gathering necessary equipment
- Traveling to golf course/driving range
- Golfing
- Returning equipment to storage
- Traveling home/to next activity

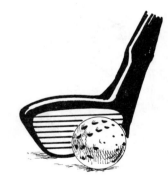

This activity requires clubs, which may be rented, borrowed, or purchased. There is usually a fee or membership requirement for play, and a specific tee time is usually scheduled. Check local public courses for their hours and prices.

All manner of clever devices are available to help players keep score.

Lessons, or supervised practice at a driving range, is strongly recommended before one takes to the fairways. You'll feel more dignified if you have *some* skill.

ITEM 1-1-16   Golfing
- a. **Driving range**
- b. **Playing the links**

Once transportation, now it's just fun!

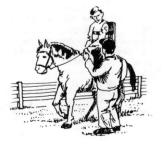

Activity includes:
- Wearing appropriate clothing
- Traveling to stable
- Riding
- Traveling home/to pickup point
- Continuing to next activity

Horseback riding can be an individual or large group activity. Fees vary from stable to stable. Charges may be for single rides or a series of lessons.

Adaptive equipment is available or can be designed for individuals who lack necessary balance. Adaptations include a modified seat or pommel, a second rider, or the use of guide horses.

It is advisable to consult with the stable director to identify a horse that will be tolerant of any modifications or rider eccentricities.

Once the rider is mounted up, the activity requires very simple motor responses.

ITEM 1-1-17   Horseback Riding

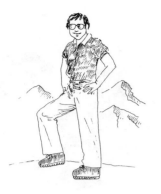

Tired of sitting all day? Get up and get out: Go take a hike!

Hiking and, if you want to be more elaborate, backpacking, are relatively easy ways to get exercise, and enjoy friends and nature. This enjoyable activity is possible in virtually any area.

Activity includes:
- Dressing in appropriate clothing
- Gathering necessary equipment
- Selecting a destination/route
- Traveling to destination
- Hiking
- Traveling home/to next activity

Participation requires a minimum of equipment and support: a good pair of shoes and a guide familiar with the terrain to be traveled. Overnight stays, of course, require more equipment and a more skillful guide.

Both the length of time required by the activity and the number of participants are flexible.

ITEM 1-1-18   Hiking/Backpacking

There have to be some *advantages to cold weather!*

Activity includes:
- Putting on appropriate outer clothing
- Gathering necessary equipment (snow-shoes, backpack, etc.)
- Traveling to site
- Putting on snowshoes
- Walking
- Changing clothes
- Returning to origin
- Returning clothes and materials to storage

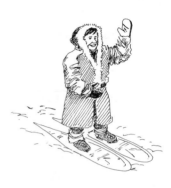

Rental equipment is available at ski shops or lodges by the day. A warm parka, mittens, and sunglasses will make the fun more comfortable.

Participation does require ability to ambulate. Speed and distance are flexible.

ITEM 1-1-19   Snowshoeing

Ski the mountains . . . or the lakes.

Skiing requires equipment and specialized clothing as well as the cooperation of Mother Nature!

Instruction and careful supervision are essential for beginners. Many winter sports areas offer specialized instruction and modified equipment for individuals with disabilities. Check with the recreation program in your community.

Activity includes:
- Gathering necessary clothing and equipment
- Traveling to ski area
- Putting on skis and other clothing as necessary
- Skiing
- Removing skis/dressing
- Traveling home/to next activity
- Returning equipment to storage

ITEM 1-1-20   Skiing
   a.   **Water skiing**   c.   **Cross country skiing**
   b.   **Downhill skiing**   d.   **Snow gourding**

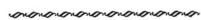

All intellectual improvement arises from leisure.
Samuel Johnson

Boating is an enjoyable way to spend a summer day.

Activity includes:
- Dressing in appropriate clothing
- Gathering necessary equipment (life-jackets, water bottle, etc.)
- Traveling to river/lake
- Preparing craft for use
- Riding/rowing/paddling
- Returning craft to storage
- Traveling home
- Returning materials to storage
- Continuing to next activity

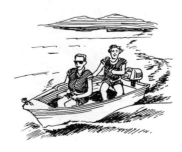

You need water for this activity . . . and a boat or water-going vessel of some sort. You may rent one or make friends with a sailor. Some community centers or park and recreation programs may rent craft or offer lessons.

Kayaks and canoes will usually require skill and participation by each rider (Note: an inactive person can ride in the front of the canoe with an experienced person paddling in the rear). Larger or motorized vessels will accommodate inactive passengers quite nicely. The routines and requirements of each craft vary considerably.

Participants should have basic water safety skills.

ITEM 1-1-21   Boating

Games/Crafts/Hobbies

Computer games are a fact of the '80s!

Most schools have a computer lab or computers available through an instructional media center. Computer games offer a great opportunity for social interaction with regular student body members. Games can be educational too! Many have been designed to practice basic academic concepts.

While the particular procedures will vary as a function of the particular brand and model of computer, in general, the activity includes:

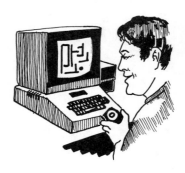

- Traveling to area
- Activating computer
- Selecting diskette with game(s) of choice
- Loading diskette
- Loading game
- Playing
- Down loading diskette
- Continuing to next activity

A picture card depicting the sequence of procedures to load/unload program makes this activity possible for most individuals.

Minimal skills are required and all levels of play are tolerated.

Responsive audio and visual displays interest many!

ITEM 1-2-1   Playing Computer Games

What Does a "Good" Goal Look Like?

Once we have selected an activity from *The Activities Catalog* to include on a person's individualized plan, we have to write it out as a goal. Writing the goal is the first step in translating an activity label into an intervention program.

A "good" goal statement specifies the target activity and describes what you expect the person to do as a result of the training or support. A "good" goal statement answers questions:

Where do I expect the person to perform? everywhere in the community or only in designated locations?

How much do I expect the person to do independently? all of it, or only certain steps while getting assistance on the others?

What steps will require modification and what kind of modification is likely?

What are other constraints or limitations I want to define?

General goals—"To improve vocational capacity," "To increase community leisure skills," or "To expand domestic competence"—really don't tell very much. A parent doesn't know what to expect. A teacher doesn't know how to design an appropriate intervention. A program manager doesn't know when important goals have been achieved.

Though it may seem complex, it is only by being clear about the intended goal that we can develop an appropriate intervention to achieve that goal.

Space Invaders! Donkey Kong! Pac Man!

What is more common these days than the whirr, blast, and bleep of the video game? It's everywhere and it's fun for children of all ages!

Video games present a great variety of sights and sounds. Play demands little strength or motor skill. The amount of time required is flexible—you can occupy a few minutes or an entire afternoon.

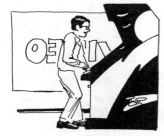

Activity includes:
- Traveling to video arcade/computer
- Selecting game
- Loading program/inserting coins
- Activating the machine
- Operating controls
- Continuing to next activity

There are important differences in coin-operated games and those games available on personal computers. Travel and expense is reduced with home play, while community visibility and social interaction are increased by play at stores, arcades, or community centers.

If you plan both computer and coin-operated play, it is important to examine the type of controls on various machines. Training machines with the same control mechanics should guarantee greatest initial success but may result in generalization problems if play expands to include still other machines.

ITEM 1-2-2   Playing Video Games
a.   On home/school computer
b.   At community location

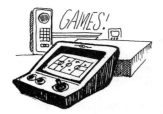

Smaller, hand-held games can go where the action is.

The student lounge, the break room, the library. Games can be played by one or two players. Though more portable than microcomputer games, hand-held videos offer less variety and less of the "status" associated with interaction with high-tech equipment.

The small visual display and relatively limited "responsiveness" may be drawbacks for some players.

This activity variation includes:

- Choosing a game
- Selecting a partner (if desired)
- Activating machine
- Playing
- Returning game to storage
- Continuing to next activity

ITEM 1-2-3   Playing Hand-Held Video Games

Portable. Flexible. Social.

Card games are an excellent way to spend a few minutes or a few hours socializing with friends.

Possible games range from simple to complex, and can be selected to match the skills of the players.

Card games present many opportunities to practice basic math skills (1:1 correspondence, numeral names, cardinal value, greater than/less than/equal) in a functional and age-appropriate context.

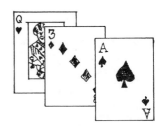

Activity includes:

- Gathering necessary materials
- Inviting others to play
- Traveling to playing area
- Dealing cards
- Playing cards as per game rules
- Re-dealing or returning materials to storage
- Continuing to next activity

Rule changes or simple devices (e.g., using a "number line" to determine the card of highest value) enable the participation of players without certain "academic" skills.

Card racks and holders, and automatic shufflers are natural modifications for players with motor difficulties.

The format is structured but flexible. It is an excellent situation to apply a variety of social skills.

ITEM 1-2-4   Playing Card Games
   a.   Regular cards
   b.   Special "game" decks (e.g., Rook, UNO)

Parchesi. Simon. Stadium Checkers.

Such games can provide a structured break during the day at school or work, or can organize an evening of fun. And the choices are mind boggling!

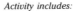

Activity includes:

- Gathering necessary game materials
- Inviting others to play
- Locating a suitable playing area
- Playing
- Returning materials to storage
- Continuing to next activity

Choose specific games. Training will then focus on the rules of a particular game rather than generic "game-playing skills."

Become thoroughly familiar with a game in order to make a judgment of its appropriateness. Games vary tremendously in their requirements for speed or academic skill. Rules can be adapted and alternate performance strategies developed. Partners play or sanctioned "kibitzing" are easy accommodations to support beginners or players who need assistance.

ITEM 1-2-5   Playing Table Games

Note: Specify target games when selecting activity.

A quiet afternoon's activity—a puzzle.
No time demands. Do it alone or with a friend.

This activity requires but two pieces of equipment: a puzzle and a table. Choose space that, once set up, can remain undisturbed.

Participation does require sight and some fine motor coordination.

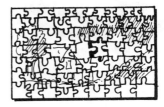

Activity includes:

- Getting puzzle
- Setting up work area
- Putting pieces together
- Cleaning up/leaving incomplete puzzle for future work
- Continuing to next activity

Take care that the subject matter depicted in the puzzle is appropriate to the chronological age of the individual. You are not doing a favor by letting an adolescent or young adult work on what is obviously a child's puzzle.

ITEM 1-2-6   Working Puzzles

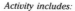

Needle crafts are an excellent way to spend a
rainy afternoon alone or in the company of friends.

Many crafts are portable and can be taken on trips or to work to occupy leisure time.

Activity includes:
- Gathering necessary materials (yarn, thread, needles, scissors, and so on)
- Locating an appropriate work area
- Working on the project
- Cleaning up work area
- Returning materials to storage
- Continuing to next activity

"Working on the project," of course, can mean many things. Most specific crafts will involve two hands, but can be adapted for individuals who have the use of only one hand. Some projects require following a pattern while others are more flexible, requiring only the repetition of a specific stitch or movement.

Cost will vary. Needles, hooks, looms, or frames are reusable. Scraps from one project can become the beginning of the next. Beginners' kits are available for most crafts, and the finishing of any project or garment can be completed by a professional or individual with more experience.

ITEM 1-2-7   Doing Needle Crafts

a.	Crocheting	d.	Spool knitting
b.	Knitting	e.	Needlepoint
c.	Embroidery	f.	Rug hooking

The most popular game in the country according to the 1980 census?
Bowling.

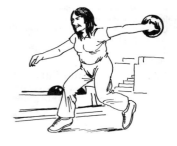

It is an ideal game for small groups or large crowds. Folks of *any* skill level have fun.

Price per game is minimal. Shoes can be rented at most bowling alleys for a nominal fee (in the range of $1). Balls are available at no charge.

Activity includes:
- Gathering money and other materials
- Traveling to bowling alley
- Renting shoes
- Putting on shoes
- Selecting ball (if necessary)
- Locating lane
- Bowling
- Returning equipment
- Paying
- Continuing to next activity

Depending on the particular location, scoring of the game may be automated. If not, players may assign responsibility to a single player, or choose a modified scoring system (estimating number of pins down, simply keeping track of balls thrown, etc.) A pocket calculator can simplify either strategy.

Alleys may have bowling ramps for players who bowl from a wheelchair and/or guide systems for players who are blind. Check to see what modifications might already be available.

ITEM 1-2-8   Bowling

- a. Tenpins
- b. Duckpins

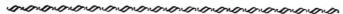

If the soul has food for study and learning, nothing is more delightful than an old age of leisure . . . . Leisure consists in all those virtuous activities by which a man grows morally, intellectually, and spiritually. It is that which makes a life worth living.

Cicero

Darts. Darts. Darts. Darts. Darts. Darts.

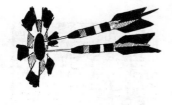

In England—and in some taverns here—this is *sport.*

You can enjoy a little "friendly competition" or simply play by and for yourself.

To the average person on the street, however, darts is a game characterized by flexibility of rules and tolerance for players of all skill levels. Scoring is optional, and many scoring variations exist (e.g., counting the number of darts that "stick" rather than the numerical value of the toss; recording individual dart values on blackboard/paper and totaling with a calculator).

Activity includes:
- Getting darts and other materials
- Inviting others to play (if desired)
- Tossing darts
- Scoring (if desired)
- Returning darts to storage
- Continuing to next activity

If the dart board is not a permanent fixture of the environment, of course an extra step will be necessary: putting up the target!

How long you play and how large the group is up to you.

ITEM 1-2-9   Playing Darts

- a. Regular darts
- b. Velcro darts

You don't have to be a "hustler" to enjoy the game.

A pool table is in the social center of many neighborhoods. Some players make money, but for most of us it's just good sport.

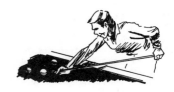

Activity includes:
- Locating pool table
- Paying for play
- Gathering necessary equipment (cues, chalk, rack, balls)

- Shooting pool
- Returning equipment
- Continuing to next activity

In pool halls or taverns, tables are rented by the hour or by the game. Home play, of course, should be free!

Game rules are flexible. Up to 8 folks can play, though interest may wane if the group gets too large.

ITEM 1-2-10   **Shooting Pool**
    a. At home
    b. At community location

Some of us have a natural talent for music . . .
*and the rest of us take **many lessons**.*

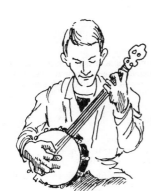

In either case, playing an instrument can structure leisure time, entertain, and provide an opportunity to collaborate with others.

Activity includes:
- Gathering instrument and necessary materials
- Going to appropriate location to play
- Preparing instrument and materials as necessary

- Playing/practicing
- Returning instrument and materials to storage
- Continuing to next activity

This activity can have major expenses: instrument purchase or rental, and lessons.

The Yellow Pages is a useful source of information. You may want to query instructors directly about their experience teaching people with disabilities.

ITEM 1-2-11   **Playing An Instrument**
    a. Piano
    b. String instrument (guitar, banjo, bass, etc.)
    c. Reed instrument (clarinet, oboe, etc.)
    d. Wind instrument (trumpet, flute, etc.)
    e. Percussion instrument (drums, cymbals, etc.)

General Case Programming

The real world is full of variation, and each activity in *The Activities Catalog* can reflect that variation.

For example, the activity "Buying Groceries" demands a slightly different performance in one store than in another across the mall. Even within the same store, the exact "shopping behaviors" can differ depending on the length of the list and the particular items to be purchased, or as a function of whether you shop at rush hour on Friday or at a low-use time during the week.

People with severe disabilities often have problems responding correctly when aspects of an activity change even slightly from the training situation. Unfortunately, for most activities it would be impossible to identify all possible variations and train in response to each alternative.

One solution to this dilemma is general case programming: a set of procedures for designing instructional programs to ensure that a person learns to perform appropriately despite situational changes. General case programming involves careful analysis of variation in circumstances and the necessary adaptations or changes in responding. Training is then carefully arranged so that the individual learns to deal with the natural changes that are expected.

If you are interested in the procedures of general case programming, we recommend several sources:

Albin, R. W., McDonnell, J. J., & Wilcox, B. (1987). Designing interventions to meet activity goals. In B. Wilcox & G. T. Bellamy, *A comprehensive guide to The Activities Catalog: An alternative curriculum for youth and adults with severe disabilities* (pp. 63–88). Baltimore: Paul H. Brookes Publishing Co.

Horner, R. H., Sprague, J. R., & Wilcox, B. (1982). General case programming for community activities. In B. Wilcox and G. T. Bellamy, *Design of high school programs for severely handicapped students* (pp. 61–98). Baltimore: Paul H. Brookes Publishing Co.

Horner, R. H., McDonnell, J. J., & Bellamy, G. T. (1986). Teaching generalized skills: General case instruction in simulation and community settings. In R. H. Horner, L. H. Meyer, & H. D. B. Fredericks (Eds.), *Education of learners with severe handicaps* (pp. 289–314). Baltimore: Paul H. Brookes Publishing Co.

A natural pack rat? Call yourself a collector and begin a hobby today!

A collection can focus on the rare or on the commonplace. Nearly anything is a collectible. Your only limits are money and space.

Expense will be affected by costs of the items to be collected and any tools or equipment necessary to organize or maintain the collection. Some collections can become a financial asset themselves!

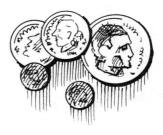

Activity includes:
- Gathering materials (items to be added, the existing collection, and any necessary tools)
- Finding an appropriate area to work
- Preparing new items

- Adding new items to collection
- Cleaning up work area
- Returning collection and materials to storage
- Continuing to next activity

Conventions or swap meets for collectors provide opportunity for social contacts as well as expanding a collection.

ITEM 1-2-12   Building a Collection

    a. **Stamps**   e. **Photos**
    b. **Coins**   f. **Comic books**
    c. **Rocks**   g. **Other**
    d. **Buttons**

Go fly a kite!

That's not an insult, but rather an invitation to a leisurely morning, afternoon, or evening. It's an opportunity to enjoy the outdoors in a way that doesn't demand speed, strength, or skill. All you really need is wind and time. Though friends—and their kites—can add to the fun, kite flying is ideal for one.

Activity includes:
- Gathering necessary materials (kite, tail, string, etc.)
- Traveling to suitable (wide-open!) location
- Launching

- Flying the kite
- Landing
- Traveling home
- Returning materials to storage
- Continuing to next activity

There are, of course, many styles of kites available and they vary considerably in cost, fragility, and maneuverability.

There is something here for everyone. A friend can provide help with the launch, and a variety of adaptations can help manage the string.

Flying model planes involves many of the same components. Equipment costs, however, are likely to be higher.

ITEM 1-2-13   Flying a Kite/Model Plane

Assessment

Assessment is the process of collecting and organizing information for decision making. In education, one of the most important decisions is what to target for training. Though we have come to equate assessment with standardized testing, we have learned that the results of those tests are not often helpful in making decisions about what is important for students to learn.

In the catalog system, assessment involves not standardized testing, but a description of an individual's life-style. Assessment asks, "What does the individual do? How often? Under what circumstances?" The result is a picture of how an individual spends his or her time.

That picture, in turn, guides decisions about how to focus instructional resources. Do we think the person would benefit by being more active? More integrated? More independent? More visible in the community? Choices about what should be taught are based on values, on what we think about the adequacy or quality of the person's life-style.

Chapter 4 in *A Comprehensive Guide to The Activities Catalog* describes how to do assessment for program planning using the catalog.

You mow the lawn so why not use it!

There are many flexible group activities that pleasantly pass an afternoon.

Activity includes:
- Gathering necessary materials/equipment
- Inviting others to play
- Locating suitable playing area
- Setting up course/equipment

- Playing
- Collecting materials
- Returning equipment to storage
- Continuing to next activity

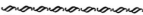
The thing that I should wish to obtain from money would be leisure with security.
               Bertrand Russell
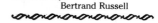

Purchase of game equipment is a one-time expense. Game rules, length of play, and team size are flexible.

ITEM 1-2-14   Playing Lawn Games

    a. **Croquet**   c. **Lawn bowling**
    b. **Jarts**   d. **Bocce ball**

Get started with a new activity or refine existing skills. How?
Go to school! A class may open the door to a lifetime of enjoyment.

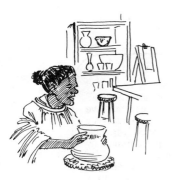

Art and craft classes are available through many sources: high schools, adult education programs, community colleges, parks and community centers, and craft shops and guilds.

Call art/craft stores or local artists for referrals or check weekly community newspapers for class schedules and fees.

Activity includes:
- Gathering necessary materials
- Locating a work station
- Working on project/following instructor
- Cleaning work area
- Continuing to next activity

By their very nature, classes include participants with all levels of skill and are relaxed and individualized, not production oriented.

Attending classes is a great way to involve neighbors or nonhandicapped friends from work or school.

ITEM 1-2-15   Attending Art/Craft Classes

a. **Ceramics**   c. **Oil Painting**
b. **Carving/Whittling** d. **Other**

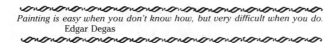

Painting is easy when you don't know how, but very difficult when you do.
Edgar Degas

Art takes many forms, and beauty is in the eye of the beholder.

These two facts open the door to a range of art projects and activities. There are countless books that suggest seasonal activities and projects that take advantage of common household items or recyclables. Both cost and complexity of the activity are flexible.

Take care to choose age-appropriate activities!

Activity includes:
- Gathering necessary materials
- Locating an appropriate work area
- Completing project
- Cleaning up work area
- Returning materials to storage
- Continuing to next activity

A self-monitoring checklist is a must for each project, especially if the type of project changes frequently. If the medium remains the same, a single generic checklist may be sufficient.

Participation typically requires some structure/assistance.

ITEM 1-2-16   Doing Miscellaneous Art Projects

Quiet but creative.

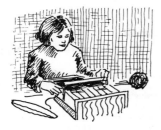

Weaving offers an opportunity to express yourself in a way that lasts.

Participation requires a loom. Once a fabric is begun it cannot be removed from the frame until completed.

Activity includes:
- Traveling to loom/work area
- Gathering necessary materials
- Weaving
- Returning materials to storage
- Continuing to next activity

There are many kinds of looms, and the style of the loom will affect the physical difficulty of the activity. Larger, more expensive models are typically more mechanized than less expensive ones. You may be able to rent a loom from a local craftsperson before making an actual purchase.

The expense of this activity will be determined primarily by the quality of yarn selected and the size of the final fabric.

There is little need to follow a pattern, for weaving is ultimately creative and flexible.

Setting up the loom and removing the completed fabric can easily be done by a more advanced weaver.

ITEM 1-2-17   Weaving/Doing Fiber Arts

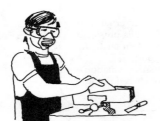

A hobby with some practical benefit.

Projects can range from cutting boards and clip boards to more elaborate pieces such as coffee tables and plant stands.

Activity includes:
- Traveling to workshop
- Gathering necessary tools and materials (safety glasses, apron, etc.)
- Working on project
- Cleaning work area
- Returning tools and material to storage
- Continuing to next activity

If tools are available, the cost of this activity will depend on the size of the project and the quality of the materials.

A tool-use fee may be charged for work done in school or community locations; check with the particular location.

ITEM 1-2-18   Woodworking
    a. At school
    b. At home
    c. At community location

Choice

Being able to make choices and control our environment—at least in part—is something we all value and take for granted. Sadly, individuals with severe handicaps often have few opportunities to make choices or control their own circumstances. Even the most basic decisions are made for them by well-intentioned parents, teachers, attendants, or friends.

How can we support choice making by people with severe handicaps? Certainly by involving them in the selection of activities for their individualized plans!

Some folks will be able to use pictures in *The Activities Catalog* to indicate interesting or preferred activities. Other individuals will be able to make selections from a smaller array of activities that are presented by a parent, teacher, or friend. For still other people, we might read off the list of activities and have them stop us when they hear activities that they might want to learn or do.

Once activities have been selected, we can be alert and offer natural choices such as where to go to lunch, what to eat, or whom to invite along to the movies. Picture cards representing the range of options can support choice-making by individuals with limited language.

You might have a green thumb. Why not give gardening a try?

Outdoor and indoor gardening each offer different rewards and challenges. Outdoor work typically involves larger plants, larger space, and full-sized tools and instruments.

Indoor gardening may involve fewer plants, in containers, and may focus more on maintenance activities. In either case, the benefits of gardening are obvious both to the gardener and to others in the home or community.

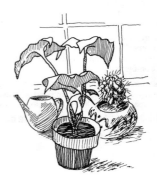

Activity includes:
- Collecting necessary tools and materials
- Going to garden area
- Completing designated tasks (watering, pruning, planting, weeding, etc.)
- Cleaning area as necessary
- Returning tools and materials to storage
- Continuing to next activity

A self-monitoring checklist can ensure that all necessary equipment is collected and that the activities are performed properly.

ITEM 1-2-19   Gardening
    a. Indoor
    b. Outdoor

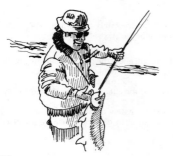

Enjoy the outdoors with friends . . . but be careful.

Fishing/hunting definitely demands both safety training and careful supervision. At the least, an error can mean injury.

Specialized equipment is required, though many items can be borrowed.

Activity includes:
- Dressing in appropriate clothing
- Gathering necessary materials and equipment
- Traveling to appropriate location
- Fishing/hunting
- Collecting materials
- Returning to point of origin
- Returning materials/equipment to storage
- Continuing to next activity

ITEM 1-2-20   Fishing/Hunting

Events

There's a club for everything: Music. Movies. Art.
Politics. Social Service. Environment. Folk Dance. Dogs. Stamps.

Club membership is an ideal way to pursue an interest and make friends with those who share it. Some clubs will have formal, structured, activity-oriented meetings. Others will be less formal and less amenable to teaching. The nature of meetings as much as the general subject matter may influence your choice of clubs.

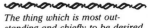
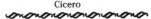

The thing which is most outstanding and chiefly to be desired by all healthy and good and well-off persons, is leisure with honour.
Cicero

Activity includes:
- Traveling to meeting location
- Participating in activities as appropriate
- Returning to next activity

Some clubs may require membership dues or activity fees.

ITEM 1-3-1   Attending Club Meetings

Note: This activity can be combined with ITEM 2-4-1: Managing a Personal Schedule.

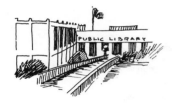

Today's library is a lot more than books. It's magazines, records, and cassettes. It's listening areas and comfy chairs. It's a place for lectures, presentations, and community affairs programs.

Going to the library is an activity for an individual, a family, or a group of friends. Time and skill requirements are flexible. There's something for everyone whether you've got a half hour or an entire afternoon.

Activity includes:
- Gathering necessary materials (library cards, books/records to be returned, etc.)
- Traveling to library
- Using library facilities (browsing, reading, listening to records/cassettes)
- Checking out materials if desired
- Traveling home/to next activity

Checking out books, tapes, or records will require a library card. Requirements for cards will depend on the community. A book bag or pack will be helpful to organize materials for transit.

ITEM 1-3-2   Using the Library

One ought, every day at least, to hear a little song, read a good poem, see a fine picture, and, if it were possible, to speak a few reasonable words.
Johann W. von Goethe

Why sit home? Pick your activity, time, and place—and GO!

Most communities offer a tremendous range of events—if you take the time to look for them. And the looking isn't hard: newspapers, radio, television, bulletin boards, and friends can tell you about more events than you could hope to attend.

Requirements for participation will depend on the event. Some may be pricey (movies, sports events, concerts). Others may have a modest admission fee (museums, fairs). Still others are free (parks, parades).

The components of participation will vary considerably as a function of the event selected. In general, however, attending a community event will include:

- Checking the time (and price!) of the event
- Dressing appropriately
- Gathering necessary materials (such as money, bus pass, or items necessary to enjoy the event)
- Traveling to the event
- Purchasing ticket if necessary
- Enjoying the event
- Traveling home/to next activity

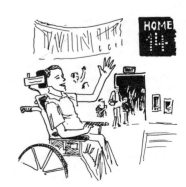

Naturally, "enjoying the event" will require different behavior for different events. Sometimes it will mean sitting quietly and listening; other times, cheering loudly for the favorite team. Though some events, such as church and movies, have fairly standard routines, many other events have minimal or very flexible structures. The key to enjoying events is having someone in the group who will highlight the demands and expectations of the particular context.

Events are often seasonal or one-time-only affairs and consequently difficult to "train." But there *is* something for everyone!

ITEM 1-3-3   Attending Community Events

a. Church
b. Movies
c. Plays/concerts/performances
d. Sports events (high school, college, semi-pro, pro, community leagues)
e. Rodeo
f. Museums
g. Exhibits and shows
h. Fairs and festivals
i. Parks
j. Parades
k. Circus
l. Parties and dances
m. Scenic rides
n. Sightseeing trips

Media

*Newspapers, magazines, and books are a common way of
getting information and keeping up to date with the world around us.*

You need *not* be a proficient reader to enjoy this activity. Just looking at pictures or scanning
the headlines is quite normal.

Activity includes:
- Selecting a paper/magazine/book
- Finding a place to sit
- Orienting the material (right side up please!)
- Looking at the material; turning pages as necessary
- Returning paper/magazine/book to original location
- Continuing to next activity

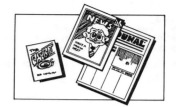

For some individuals, training may focus on locating sections or information of interest (e.g.,
sports, weather, leisure events).

There are many opportunities to use this activity: at home, in the school or community library,
in the doctor's waiting room, or in the break room. Time is flexible and cost minimal.

This can be an excellent way to respond to an individual's special interest areas.

ITEM 1-4-1   Reading Newspapers/Magazines/Books

*Note: This activity can be nicely combined with ITEM 1-3-2: Using the Library, and reading
materials can be purchased as part of ITEM 2-3-1: Purchasing Personal Items.*

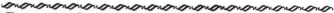

*The newspapers! Sir, they are the most villainous—licentious—abominable—
informal—not that I ever read them—no—I make it a rule never to look into a
newspaper.*
 Richard B. Sheridan

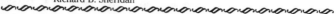

*What would life be without music?
Or news? Don't force yourself to find out.*

The radio is a readily available and inexpensive form of entertainment.

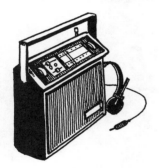

Activity includes:
- Locating radio
- Turning on equipment
- Adjusting the volume
- Selecting a station
- Listening to program
- Turning off equipment
- Returning radio to storage
- Continuing to next activity

Participation requires a radio—nothing more! And there is no limit on how long you can enjoy
listening!

A small portable radio with headphones may be used to eliminate the monotony of work or
exercise routines.

ITEM 1-4-2   Listening to the Radio

Music without the worry of records! Part of today's youth culture.

Activity includes:
- Locating cassette player
- Selecting a tape
- Inserting tape
- Turning on player
- Listening to program
- Changing tape as necessary/desired
- Turning off player
- Returning tape(s) and player to storage
- Continuing to next activity

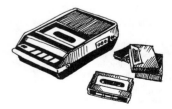

All you need is a collection of tapes and a tape player. Players come in various formats, many of
which are portable.

ITEM 1-4-3   Using a Cassette Player

Reading without books—enjoy a good story without straining your eyes!

You can be entertained by a good story while walking, riding in a car, or just relaxing.

This variation of using a tape player is available simply by purchasing books on tape rather
than music.

These cassettes are available at bookstores or from the American Printing House for the Blind,
1839 Frankfurt Ave., Louisville, KY 40206   (502) 895-2406.

Books on tape and tape players are also available free of charge to qualified individuals
through the Library of Congress, Library for the Blind and Physically Handicapped. Check your
phone book for a local branch.

*Some men are so selfish that they
read a book or go to a concert for
their own sinister pleasure, instead
of doing it to improve social conditions, as the good citizen does
when drinking cocktails or playing
bridge.*

 Jacques Barzun

ITEM 1-4-4   Listening to Talking Books

*Note: Individuals who enjoy playing records or tapes may want to consider related activities such
as checking out records or tapes from the library (ITEM 1-3-2: Using the Library) or buying
additional records or tapes (ITEM 2-3-1: Purchasing Personal Items).*

A possibility for home, school, or break time at work!

Listening to records is a flexible, individual activity.

Activity includes:

- Locating records and record player/ stereo
- Selecting a record
- Putting record on record player
- Turning on record player
- Adjusting volume

- Listening
- Removing record
- Selecting a different record as desired
- Turning off record player
- Returning records to storage
- Proceeding to next activity

Activity requires a record player/stereo and a selection of records.
Time requirements are flexible: you can listen as long as you can listen.
Common modifications include headphones that permit user enjoyment without infringing on the airwaves of others in the environment.

ITEM 1-4-5   Playing Records

Life can't be all bad when for ten dollars you can buy all the Beethoven sonatas and listen to them for ten years.
William F. Buckley, Jr.

Bring the movies home! And bring friends from school or the workplace along!

Showing a good movie at home provides a natural opportunity for supervised interaction with nonhandicapped friends and is an easy way to maintain social contacts.
Primarily an activity for the home, using a video cassette recorder (VCR) includes:

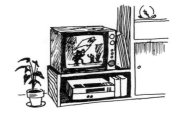

- Selecting a movie cassette
- Locating the VCR
- Turning on player
- Inserting cassette
- Adjusting volume

- Watching
- Ejecting cassette
- Turning off equipment
- Continuing to next activity

VCRs are available for rent at many local outlets.

ITEM 1-4-6   Using a VCR

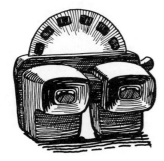

The world at your fingertips! This is a perfect passive leisure activity for the individual who enjoys visual stimulation.

For the price of a viewmaster and individual cartridges you can see the world . . . or view other interesting subject matter.

Activity includes:

- Getting viewmaster and cartridges
- Inserting cartridge
- Viewing pictures

- Changing the cartridge as desired
- Returning materials to storage
- Continuing to next activity

Participation requires relatively simple motor responses.

ITEM 1-4-7   Using a Viewmaster

I find television very educating. Every time somebody turns on the set I go into the other room and read a book.
Groucho Marx

You may not like it but it's here to stay: the television.

Activity includes:

- Locating set
- Turning on set
- Adjusting volume
- Selecting program

- Watching program
- Turning off set
- Continuing to next activity

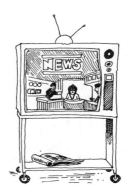

Obviously you can't proceed without a television!
Fortunately for others in the environment, some models do have earphones!
While some individuals may select programs using the regular TV guide, others may need adapted and individualized timetables that depict favorite shows, times, and stations.

ITEM 1-4-8   Watching Television

Other

Reach out and touch someone.

Not a bad idea. Calling nearby friends or family is an easy, inexpensive way to stay in touch, make plans, or relieve the boredom of the moment.

The activity of *making calls* includes:

- Locating telephone
- Dialing number
- Saying hello/requesting target person
- Talking/leaving message
- Saying goodbye
- Hanging up
- Continuing to next activty

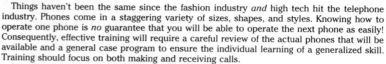

Things haven't been the same since the fashion industry *and* high tech hit the telephone industry. Phones come in a staggering variety of sizes, shapes, and styles. Knowing how to operate one phone is *no* guarantee that you will be able to operate the next phone as easily! Consequently, effective training will require a careful review of the actual phones that will be available and a general case program to ensure the individual learning of a generalized skill. Training should focus on both making and receiving calls.

A personalized picture directory of frequently called people and numbers will eliminate the need to remember numbers or to struggle with the phone book.

The activity of *receiving calls* includes:

- Locating phone
- Picking up receiver
- Saying hello
- Responding to caller
- Saying goodbye
- Hanging up
- Continuing to next activty

There are many different ways of taking a message if a caller asks for someone who is not available to come to the phone. Strategies include writing from dictation, using a check-off form similar to those in use in many offices, turning on a tape recorder to record the message, or simply instructing the caller to "call again, please." The strategy should be determined prior to beginning training, and should, of course, consider individual skills and the preferences of the household.

ITEM 1-5-1 **Talking with Friends/Family on the Telephone**
   a. **Making calls**
   b. **Receiving calls**

Note: For further information, see Horner, R. H., Williams, J. A., & Steveley, J. D. (in press). Acquisition of generalized telephone use by students with severe mental retardation. *Journal of Applied Research in Mental Retardation.*

There are friends . . . and lovers.

Intimacy is important to all of us. Developing those special relationships takes time . . . and a certain amount of luck.

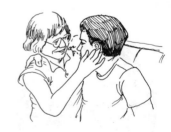

It's not something we can teach. The best we can do is provide opportunity. Simply doing things together is important. Belonging to a club, eating dinner, attending sporting events, or sharing a hobby can all build the base for a relationship. Physical intimacy may be a natural result.

Supporting intimate relationships may require explicit information and instruction about sexual expression and birth control. Most certainly it requires the opportunity to make a choice. Since intimate relationships may represent situations where the wishes of an individual with severe disabilities may conflict with those of his or her parents, it may be important to involve a third-party advocate.

ITEM 1-5-2 **Maintaining Intimate Relationships**

Liberty is being free from the things we don't like in order to be slaves of the things we do like.
   Ernest Benn

A stroll down the block. A cross-country flight.
Do what it takes to keep in touch with family and friends.

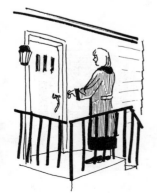

In today's mobile society it takes effort and planning to maintain the social network that is so vital to each one of us. Visiting is a way to reach out, to expand horizons, to be on our own. Visits away from home are an important step in growing up.

Activity includes:

- Making arrangements for visit (establishing date, time, means of transportation, etc.)
- Gathering necessary materials (e.g., clothing, money, gifts)
- Traveling to target home/location
- Visiting
- Traveling home/to next activity

Naturally, transportation to and from visits can often be provided by family or friends, thus eliminating the need to train walking or bus routes. When walking or mass transit are the method of choice, sequenced picture cards can provide a clear reminder of the correct route. For long-distance trips by bus, train, or plane, preparations will be more extensive and more detailed provisions made to ensure supervision and assistance as necessary along the way.

ITEM 1-5-3 **Visiting Family/Friends**

Developing Friendships

Friends are important to all of us. We each know that we just can't make it alone. We need the assistance, encouragement, and love of family, spouse, or friends. Individuals with disabilities are no exceptions.

Unfortunately, individuals with disabilities often have limited social networks. Their contacts are too often limited to other people with disabilities or to people who are paid caregivers (teachers, aides, group home providers, or attendants). Individualized planning meetings provide a natural time to think about what we can do to help people with disabilities make friends and expand that important social network.

The research literature on friendship has identified several factors that influence whether people become friends.

1. *Opportunities to interact.* Obviously folks can't very well become friends unless they have regular opportunities to interact and get to know each other. By selecting activity goals that put people with disabilities in regular contact with a social group, you are helping to build the basis for friendships.
2. *Image of similarity.* People are more likely to develop friendships with others who have shared interests and experiences. Selecting activities that are age appropriate and that take advantage of the opportunities available in a community highlights similarities between a person with a severe disability and his or her nonhandicapped peers. Doing things together builds a shared history and demonstrates shared interests.
3. *Competence.* People are more likely to become friends when they have the skills to initiate and sustain interactions. Concentrating on the social components of target activities will help build social competence for future encounters. In addition, having something to do together—going to a sporting event or to the corner café for coffee and a donut—represents another important form of competence basic to friendships.

Friendships don't develop in a vacuum but in the context of daily activities. While "having friends" is not an activity you can order from *The Activities Catalog,* you can increase the probability of friendships through the selection of activities that will provide the context.

If you are interested in a description of the kind of friendships that are possible between individuals with severe disabilities and folks without apparent handicaps, see the article entitled "Friendships and Our Children" by Jeff and Cindy Strully in the *Journal of the Association for Persons with Severe Handicaps* (1985, *16,* pp. 224–227).

Sauna. Hot Tub. Whirlpool. Steam Room.

Once hard to find, these methods of relaxation are now common features in most gymnasiums, health clubs, and YMCAs.

Time in a spa is a great way to finish off a hard day of work or a well-fought game. Nothing, but nothing, erases the cares of the day or eases tired muscles like heat.

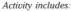

Activity includes:

- Gathering necessary materials (towel, suit, pass, etc.)
- Traveling to whirlpool/steamroom/sauna/hot tub
- Locating locker room/changing area
- Changing out of street clothes (and into suit or towel as desired/as appropriate)
- Using whirlpool/steam room/hot tub/sauna
- Showering
- Changing into street clothes
- Gathering materials
- Traveling home/to next activity

Access to spas may require club memberships or fees. Prices will vary. Call ahead to determine hours, cost, and whether towels and lockers are provided.

ITEM 1-5-4   **Using a Whirlpool/Steam Room/Hot Tub/Sauna**

Get a perfect tan with—or without—the sun!

No doubt about it. A tan makes you look and feel good. And with today's technology, there's no reason to be pale. But don't overdo it!

Sunbathing is free . . . but requires the cooperation of the weather. Using a tanning salon ensures sun when *you* want it. The cost of tanning sessions will vary. Single sessions and packages are available. Call around to get the best price.

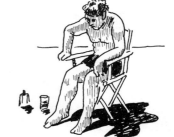

Activity includes:

- Gathering necessary materials (towel, sunglasses, and sunscreen)
- Traveling to salon/pool/appropriate location
- Changing out of street clothes (and into suit)
- Tanning
- Changing into street clothes
- Traveling home/to next activity

Spas or salons will supervise the length of the tanning sessions, and will often supply towels, sunscreens, and moisturizers.

ITEM 1-5-5   **Using a Tanning Salon/Sunbathing**

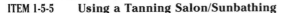

Dance the night away!

It's a nice way to meet friends, have fun, and get some exercise, too.

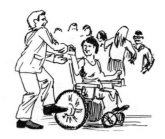

Activity includes:
- Dressing in appropriate clothing
- Gathering necessary materials (money, identification, etc.)
- Traveling to dance hall
- Dancing/relaxing
- Traveling home/to next activity

What do you need for dancing? Shoes and a partner! Beyond that, the cost for an evening will depend on the establishment. A cover charge is common, so be prepared. Go alone, with a partner, or as a group.

Assistance may be necessary to identify dress appropriate to the style of dancing or the particular establishment. It is best to call ahead to see if there are restrictions on shoes or dress.

ITEM 1-5-6   Going out Dancing

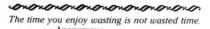
The time you enjoy wasting is not wasted time.
Anonymous
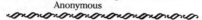

The local pub.

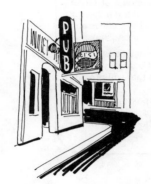

A social institution in many communities. Drop by for a quick stop or for a longer evening. A place to meet or make friends.

Activity includes:
- Preparing to go (checking appearance; getting money and identification; etc.)
- Traveling to bar/tavern
- Ordering food/beverage
- Drinking/relaxing
- Returning home/to next activity

Bars and taverns often offer much more than a drink. They frequently have big screen television, music, darts, pool, pinball, or dancing.

Of course, use good judgment in selecting a drinking establishment! If drinking is a worry, you can manage the quantity consumed by sending along a friend, by restricting the amount of money taken, by prior arrangement with the bartender or waitress, or by ordering nonalcoholic beverages.

As always, there should be a variety of ways to arrange transportation, depending on the location of the bar/tavern.

ITEM 1-5-7   Going to a Bar/Tavern

Note: This activity can be combined with ITEM 2-1-1: Using Restrooms.

Personal Management

There is simply no way to get around the need to use a restroom.

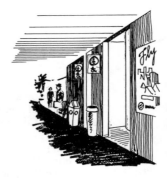

Activity includes:
- Recognizing need
- Locating bathroom
- Adjusting clothing
- Voiding
- Wiping
- Adjusting clothing
- Washing hands
- Returning to ongoing/next activity

There is great variation in how restrooms are labeled (Men/Women, Boys/Girls, Braves/Squaws, or no label at all!), how they are laid out, and how toilet, soap and paper dispensers, and faucets operate. Be sure that training matches the requirements of those restrooms that the person will actually use.

ITEM 2-1-1   **Using Restrooms**
        a.   Home
        b.   School/work
        c.   Public

Note: This item can be combined with most community leisure activities.

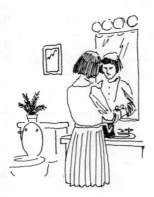

For Women Only.

For about 3–7 days each month, all women need to care for their menstrual hygiene.

Given the range of available products, the family, an advocate, or the planning team should give thought to the general style and particular brand that would be most appropriate for each individual. Training can then be product specific.

Activity includes:
- Locating necessary materials
- Traveling to bathroom or private area
- Removing undergarments
- Removing used pantyliner/pad/tampon
- Replacing pantyliner/pad/tampon
- Disposing appropriately of wrapper/ other garbage
- Adjusting clothing
- Continuing to ongoing/next activity.

Competence in this activity will be facilitated if the onset and duration of each menstrual cycle is recorded on a personal calendar. This allows the individual, family members, care providers, or advocates to anticipate the need, ensure the availability of supplies, provide review, and ensure that training resources are available as necessary.

Conservative planning would suggest that the individual always carry tampons/pads in her purse and have a supply available at school or work.

ITEM 2-1-2   **Taking Care of Menstrual Needs**

Note: This can be coordinated with ITEM 2-3-1: Purchasing Personal Items.

Having stylish hair helps us look and feel our best.

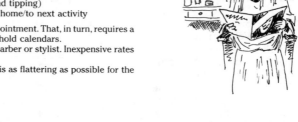

Getting a haircut is not a frequent activity—perhaps once every 4–8 weeks—but it is one that highlights our individuality.

Activity includes:
- Making and recording appointment
- Preparing to go (checking appearance, getting money, etc.)
- Traveling to barber/beauty salon
- Announcing arrival
- Waiting while hair is washed/cut/styled
- Paying (and tipping)
- Returning home/to next activity

Typically, getting one's hair cut or styled will require an appointment. That, in turn, requires a system for recording the appointment on personal or household calendars.

The cost of this activity will depend on the charges of the barber or stylist. Inexpensive rates may be available through barber or beauty colleges.

Do check with the stylist to ensure that the particular cut is as flattering as possible for the target individual.

ITEM 2-1-3   **Getting Hair Cut/Styled**

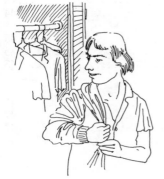

There is quite simply no getting around this one: You must get dressed.

In what you wear and how you get it on, of course, there is tremendous variability.

Activity includes:
- Selecting appropriate clothing items
- Putting on undergarments
- Putting on outer garments
- Putting on footwear
- Continuing to next activity

Some of us take the worry out of clothing selection by relying on a standard set of outfits (*always* wear the gray skirt, pink blouse, and navy sweater together) or by creating a wardrobe where all items are interchangeable. These strategies are equally helpful to people with disabilities. Acceptable outfits can be hung together in the closet or photographed and included in a "what to wear?" file on the dresser.

Consider whether there are styles of garments or types of closures that will support greater independence by the particular person.

There are a myriad of devices that assist people with physical limitations or disabilities to dress themselves.

ITEM 2-1-4   **Dressing**

What goes on must come off . . . at some point.

Activity includes:
- Going to private/appropriate area
- Removing shoes
- Removing outer garments
- Removing undergarments
- Placing items in designated location (closet, clothes hamper)

- Putting on nightwear/next set of garments
- Continuing to next activity

ITEM 2-1-5   Undressing

Note: Many activities include changing from one type of clothing into another (e.g., swimming includes changing from street clothes to a swimsuit/trunks and back again). As a consequence, dressing and undressing may be coordinated with any or all such activities. For training, more detailed task analyses may be necessary for each garment type.

No two people begin the day alike—but everyone begins the day.

Structuring your morning routine is one of the ways that you fit into the household routine and express your own individuality. Whether you are "a 5-minute beauty" or require 45 minutes to become presentable, there is still a routine.

Except for a small number of elements that seem culturally prescribed, there is great flexibility in getting ready for the day. Choose those elements that match your style. Others can be included in the evening routine and some can be overlooked altogether!

Brushing teeth is something you probably can't avoid. The nature of the task, though, will vary depending on whether you choose a standard or electric toothbrush.
Includes:
- Arranging necessary materials (brush, toothpaste, glass)
- Applying paste to brush
- Brushing teeth
- Rinsing mouth

- Rinsing brush and glass
- Returning materials to storage
- Continuing to next activity/element of morning routine

Pump toothpaste dispensers or inverted tubes with "keys" are modifications that simplify motor and coordination demands for some individuals, as does an electric toothbrush.

Using deodorant/antiperspirant is another "must."
Includes:
- Locating deodorant/antiperspirant
- Removing cap/top
- Applying to underarm
- Replacing cap

- Returning container to storage
- Continuing to next activity/element of morning routine

Shaving is a daily event for most men. If you decide not to grow a beard, the major decision that structures this element is whether to use an electric or a safety razor.
Using an electric razor includes:
- Gathering materials (shaver, aftershave lotion)
- Turning on shaver
- Shaving
- Turning off shaver

- Cleaning equipment
- Applying aftershave lotion
- Returning materials to storage
- Continuing to next activity/element of morning routine

Using a safety razor includes:
- Gathering necessary materials (razor, shaving cream or soap)
- Lathering beard
- Shaving
- Rinsing off razor

- Rinsing face
- Returning materials to storage
- Continuing to next activity/element of morning routine

Taking a bath includes:
- Gathering necessary materials (soap, towel)
- Undressing
- Turning on water
- Adjusting water temperature
- Closing tub drain
- Filling tub

- Turning off water
- Entering tub
- Washing and rinsing off
- Releasing stopper
- Toweling dry
- Continuing to next activity/element of morning routine

Taking a shower includes:
- Gathering necessary materials (soap, towel)
- Undressing
- Turning on water
- Adjusting water temperature
- Entering shower

- Washing and rinsing off
- Turning off water
- Toweling dry
- Continuing to next activity/element of morning routine

Be sure to note the style of fixture so that instruction fits the operation of the particular fixture.

Washing face and hands is usually included as an element of the *morning* routine if bathing/ showering is defined as part of the *evening* routine.
Includes:

- Gathering necessary equipment (wash-cloth, soap, towel)
- Turning on water
- Adjusting water temperature
- Wetting and soaping cloth
- Washing face
- Rinsing
- Drying face
- Returning materials to storage location
- Continuing to next element of morning routine

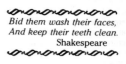
Washing hair is most easily included with a shower or bath but may be done separately if facilities allow. The planning team should make this decision along with a determination of frequency with which this element should be performed.
Includes:

- Gathering necessary materials (shampoo, conditioner, towel, comb)
- Turning on water
- Adjusting water flow and temperature
- Wetting hair
- Shampooing hair
- Rinsing hair
- Conditioning hair
- Rinsing hair
- Turning off water
- Toweling dry
- Combing out hair
- Returning materials to storage
- Continuing to next activity/element of morning routine

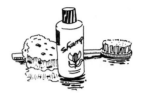

Blow drying hair depends on your preference for style! Begins with wet hair.
Includes:

- Gathering necessary materials (dryer, comb, brush)
- Turning on dryer
- Drying and combing hair to desired dryness
- Turning off dryer
- Returning materials to storage
- Continuing to next element of morning routine

Using rollers/curling iron/etc. usually begins with hair that is dry or blown dry. Success requires some plan for setting the rollers or applying the curling iron.
Includes:

- Gathering necessary materials (rollers/curling iron, comb, fasteners, etc.)
- Turning on equipment
- Combing hair
- Rolling hair on curlers or curling iron
- Removing rollers or iron
- Turning off/unplugging rollers or iron
- Combing out
- Returning materials to storage
- Continuing to next element of morning routine

There are many types and styles of curling and rolling equipment, some quite easy to use and others more difficult. Be sure to consider the motor and coordination demands of the individual before purchasing equipment.

Flossing, which every dentist considers "a must," would usually follow brushing the teeth.
Includes:

- Obtaining floss
- Cutting length of floss
- Flossing between teeth
- Discarding floss
- Returning floss container to storage
- Continuing to next activity/element of morning routine.

Using mouthwash may lead to romance as the commercials promise or it may simply be a refreshing way to begin the day. It would usually follow brushing teeth.
Includes:

- Gathering necessary materials (mouthwash, glass)
- Pouring mouthwash into glass
- Gargling
- Rinsing
- Returning materials to storage
- Continuing to next activity/element of morning routine

Using cologne/perfume/powder is a matter of taste. Choose a suitable fragrance, perhaps with advice from others. And don't clash with yourself! This is a final touch to the morning routine.
Includes:

- Locating cologne/powder
- Applying as appropriate
- Returning material to storage
- Continuing to next activity/element of morning routine

Examine the container carefully for modifications to facilitate use. It may be quite possible to leave a shaker open or a top off.

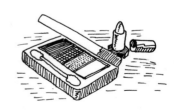

Using makeup can highlight your appearance and help keep you in style. The choice of colors should be made with advice from others. Such assistance is routinely available at cosmetic counters in major department stores or through beauty salons.

Shaving legs and underarms is a frequent/daily event for most women. It can be done with an electric or safety razor. If the choice is to use a safety razor, the task is naturally combined with bath or shower; if an electric razor is available, the task can be done at any time.
Includes:

- Gathering materials (shaver, after-shave)
- Turning on shaver
- Shaving
- Turning off shaver
- Cleaning equipment
- Returning materials to storage
- Continuing to next activity/element of morning routine.

Caring for dirty clothing items will be structured by the larger household routine. Individuals may be asked to put dirty clothes in a laundry bag in their own room or to deposit them in a central hamper in the bathroom or a laundry area.

The material and equipment requirements of this activity will depend on the particular elements selected. There is a tremendous range in product packaging and equipment style that may affect individual performance, so consider options carefully before making a choice.

A picture self-monitoring system is helpful in defining the elements of the morning routine and sequencing them for logical completion.

ITEM 2-1-6　Completing Morning Routine

a.	Brushing teeth	i.	Using rollers/curling iron/etc.
b.	Using deodorant/anti-perspirant	k.	Using mouthwash
c.	Shaving	l.	Using cologne/perfume/powder
d.	Taking a bath	m.	Using makeup
e.	Taking a shower	n.	Shaving legs and under-arms
f.	Washing face and hands	o.	Caring for dirty clothing
g.	Washing hair		
h.	Blow drying hair		
j.	Flossing		

Note: This activity may be coordinated with ITEM 2-3-1: Purchasing Personal Items. The planning team should review this activity and ITEM 2-1-7: Completing Evening Routine to ensure that all necessary personal hygiene elements are included in one activity or the other.

As each day begins, so it must end.

There is a tremendous variation in evening routine. Choose elements that were not included in the morning routine or those that make sense to repeat because of preference or personal hygiene needs.

Use picture self-monitoring cards to define and structure the routine.

ITEM 2-1-7　Completing Evening Routine may include:

a.	Brushing teeth	g.	Flossing
b.	Using deodorant/antiperspirant	h.	Using rollers/curling iron/etc.
c.	Taking a bath	i.	Shaving legs and underarms
d.	Taking a shower	j.	Caring for dirty clothing
e.	Washing hair		
f.	Blow drying hair		

Good Simulations

Simulations—training in a situation that is not the natural environment—can be used to provide extra practice on difficult steps of an activity or to provide more control for a trainer than would be possible in the natural setting itself.

The effectiveness of a simulation should always be judged by how well it improves performance in the natural environment.

Good simulations: 1) incorporate the same stimuli that should control behavior in the natural environment, 2) have the person practice a response that is similar in form to the response required in the natural setting, and 3) are always combined with training in at least one natural setting.

For more information about designing simulations, see:

Albin, R. W., McDonnell, J. J., & Wilcox, B. (1987). Designing interventions to meet activity goals. In B. Wilcox & G. T. Bellamy, *A comprehensive guide to The Activities Catalog: An alternative curriculum for youth and adults with severe disabilities* (pp. 63–88). Baltimore: Paul H. Brookes Publishing Co.

Food

Don't feel like cooking? Enjoy a quick meal out.

Fast-food restaurants have become part of our way of life. Once limited to hamburgers, shakes, and fries, fast-food establishments now offer an astonishing array of cuisines. They offer breakfast, lunch, and dinner—and, of course, snacks.

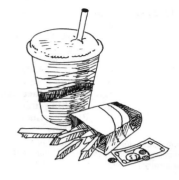

Activity includes:

- Preparing to go (checking appearance; getting money and other necessary materials)
- Traveling to restaurant
- Entering
- Placing the order
- Paying for purchase
- Carrying food to empty table
- Eating
- Cleaning up
- Traveling home/to next activity

Fast-food restaurants are *everywhere* . . . and they are different. You will need to decide which restaurants and which locations will be used. It will be necessary to devise a system for travel to each location, and to differentiate where one might walk or would need to be driven. The order of the routine may vary (in one you may get food and then pay while in another the order is reversed), so it is important that the trainer be familiar with the training sites.

It is desirable to maximize choice in this activity by devising a strategy that permits the individual to select the particular restaurant and his or her own meal. Several ways to adapt difficult steps of this activity support the participation of people with disabilities:

Use *menu cards* that picture the individual items available at the restaurant and their cost (rounded up to include tax if applicable).

Use a calculator and a *"Can I Afford It?"* strategy for budgeting. The cost of the target meal can be added up and the necessary amount of money packaged prior to leaving for the restaurant. The menu cards themselves can double as communication cards in the restaurant.

Use a *next-dollar* strategy to pay for the purchase.

ITEM 2-2-1   Using Fast-Food Restaurants

Dining out. One of life's pleasures . . . and something we have come to associate with quality of life.

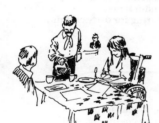

Activity includes:

- Preparing to go (checking appearance; gathering necessary materials; selecting restaurant; and so on)
- Traveling to restaurant
- Entering
- Waiting to be seated
- Ordering
- Eating
- Paying for meal (and tipping!)
- Traveling home/to next activity

Reservations are necessary at many restaurants, so it is important to know your dining establishments! If reservations are made in advance, it will be necessary to record the date/time on the individual's schedule or self-monitoring system.

Unlike fast-food establishments, patrons of sit-down restaurants are expected to leave a tip, so some strategy will be necessary to determine the size of the tip. Asking another patron to suggest an amount or requesting that the waiter compute a 15% gratuity on the bill are but two alternatives.

Establishing the particular restaurants an individual is to patronize regularly makes it possible to develop training materials to facilitate choice and budgeting.

ITEM 2-2-2   Using a Sit-Down Restaurant

Note: This activity can be combined with ITEM 2-1-1: Using Restrooms.

Somewhere between fast food and four-star food is the cafeteria.

The cafeteria is an establishment in most schools and many businesses. If cafeteria-style eateries are commonplace in your community, it might be wise to know their rules!

Activity includes:

- Preparing to go (checking appearance; getting money and other necessary materials)
- Traveling to cafeteria
- Joining end of the line
- Getting a tray, utensils, and other materials
- Selecting food items
- Paying for purchases
- Transporting tray to table
- Eating
- Cleaning up
- Traveling home/to next activity

Eat, drink and be merry,
for tomorrow ye diet.
Lewis C. Henry

Perhaps the greatest danger of a cafeteria is selecting more than you can eat . . . or pay for! This can be handled by using menu cards to select items in advance from an array of items available, or by using a calculator and a cumulative subtraction strategy as you move through the line.

Those individuals who have difficulty carrying a tray will need a clear system for requesting assistance.

ITEM 2-2-3   Using a Cafeteria

***Who would have imagined the day when humans would
derive a substantial part of their sustenance from machines?***

Competence with vending machines is almost a requirement of modern civilization. Certainly no adolescent can live without it!

Activity includes:
- Locating vending machine
- Inserting coins
- Activating machine
- Securing item
- Checking for change
- Consuming item purchased
- Continuing to next activity

Participation requires money, and choice may be restricted by funds available.

Problems with coin skills? Consider developing index cards that picture an item/logo on the front and depict the price with coin stamps on the back. Then by matching coins to the coin stamps, a person can choose an item and determine the necessary coins in advance. Or consider a strategy that simply teaches the user to deposit four quarters (and of course check for change). That strategy will work for many items . . . at least until inflation sets in!

Since there is tremendous variation across vending machines, it is important either to identify specific machines that will be used in training or to develop an instructional program that teaches the general case.

ITEM 2-2-4   Using Vending Machines

Note: For further information, see Sprague, J., & Horner, R. (1984). The effects of single instance, multiple instance and general case training on generalized vending machine use by moderately and severely handicapped students. *Journal of Applied Behavior Analysis, 17,* 273–278.

***Since at school, at work, or at play you may find yourself face-to-face
with a snack bar, it might not be a bad idea to know how to use it!***

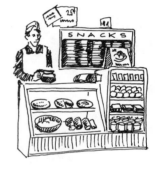

The cost of this activity can be adjusted for most any budget since snack bars typically offer an array of inexpensive items.

Activity includes:
- Traveling to snack bar
- Placing order
- Paying for purchase
- Eating
- Disposing of trash appropriately
- Returning to next activity

Preselecting items, using picture communication cards, and using overpayment strategies can help individuals without academic skills be successful at this activity.

ITEM 2-2-5   Using a Snack Shop/Canteen

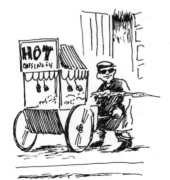

***Big cities. Campuses. Parks. And—of course—sporting events. These are
the places you are likely to find street vendors with their assortment of
treats. Soft pretzels and mustard. Hot dogs. Ice cream bars. Smoothies.
Cotton candy. These are some of the delights available from "the wagon."***

If yours is an area where vendors are common, you should learn to deal with them.

Activity includes:
- Approaching vendor
- Ordering
- Paying for item
- Eating
- Disposing of trash appropriately
- Continuing to next activity

Communication cards and "prepackaged" money can facilitate this activity for many individuals.

ITEM 2-2-6   Using Street Vendors

It All Sounds Nice But What If the System Isn't Responsive?

You like the idea of targeting natural activities for your son or daughter . . . but you know the system won't. Don't be discouraged. Change is always a difficult process.

If you find yourself on your own without the support of the educational or human services system, you may want to try some of the life-style planning strategies described by John O'Brien in *A comprehensive guide to The Activities Catalog: An alternative curriculum for youth and adults with severe disabilities* (Wilcox & Bellamy, 1987, pp. 175–189). He offers useful suggestions for an informal planning process when the formal process does not seem to meet your needs.

Somebody has to do it—if you want to eat, that is!

Shopping for groceries is basic to the maintenance of most households. It may be done weekly or daily. An individual may be responsible for the entire list or only a subset of items. There is no cost to this activity—other than the cost of the groceries themselves.

Activity includes:

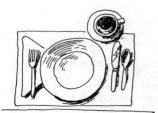

- Preparing to go (checking appearance; getting money, shopping list, and other materials)
- Traveling to store
- Entering
- Getting cart

- Selecting items (locating aisle, locating item)
- Locating checkout counters
- Paying for items
- Collecting groceries
- Returning home/to next activity

Competent performance of this activity will require decisions regarding:

- The particular stores in which the individual will be expected to shop after training
- The length of the grocery list (viz., the number of items that will be purchased)

- Whether purchases are to be brand and size specific
- The strategy that will be used to pay for items (charge account, next-dollar strategy, etc.)

Decisions to shop in multiple locations, to shop for a large range of items, or to use a "next-dollar" payment strategy all suggest the need for a general case instructional program.

Individuals with motor problems or with limited strength or stamina may need adaptations to remove items from shelves or to transport items from the store.

In most households, it will also be necessary to devise a strategy for scheduling grocery shopping.

ITEM 2-2-7   Buying Groceries

Note: This activity can be coordinated with ITEM 2-2-10: Planning Meals and ITEM 2-2-8: Storing Groceries.

Once the groceries are home, there's still work to be done—they must be put away.

Activity includes:

- Unpacking bags/boxes
- Opening cupboards/storage areas
- Placing items in designated areas

- Closing cupboards/storage areas
- Disposing of or putting away bags/boxes
- Continuing to next activity

For people without the skill to classify items, this activity may be done with a partner who designates the target location for each product.

ITEM 2-2-8   Storing Groceries

Note: This activity can be combined with ITEM 2-2-7: Buying Groceries.

It's a chore that doesn't go away when you grow up.
And it's one that has to be done if you're to qualify as "civilized."

Setting the table will occur routinely at the evening meal and at other meals depending on the life-style of the household. It is a regular chore and consequently an easy way for an individual to make a regular contribution.

Activity includes:

- Clearing or cleaning eating areas as necessary
- Determining number of place settings needed

- Gathering necessary materials (silverware, glasses, plates, and so on)
- Positioning items appropriately
- Continuing to next activity

Establishing a fixed routine can make this activity easy for almost anyone. A self-monitoring card that pictures each step of the process and each type of item in the place setting eliminates the need for memory or judgment. The number of places to be set can be standardized or designated separately for each meal.

ITEM 2-2-9   Setting the Table

What's for dinner? Or lunch? Or breakfast?

Meal planning occurs as part of a larger system of food management designed for an individual or for a household.

Meal planning can take many forms, depending on that system. It can be so elaborate that it requires the skills of a licensed dietitian or it can be as simple as pulling a picture menu and recipe cards from a file of "balanced meals." Meal planning can be done each day or for an entire week or month. As items are used up, there must be a strategy to add them to the shopping list.

Systems should be devised with the collaboration of parents, teachers, or advocates. The development of picture menu and recipe cards, picture grocery shopping cards, coded systems for monitoring the availability of ingredients, and so on, all will require some external support.

To maximize choice and independence, we suggest a system that relies on a limited set of menus developed by a parent, teacher, or advocate.

Relying on prepared foods rather than "cooking from scratch" may be somewhat more expensive but controls portions and promotes greater independence.

Care, of course, should be taken to ensure that the standard menus developed are indeed nutritionally balanced and responsive to the preferences of the individual(s).

ITEM 2-2-10   Planning Meals

Note: This activity should be coordinated with ITEM 2-2-7: Buying Groceries.

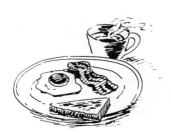

Once a meal is planned, there is still work to be done!

Activity includes:
- Selecting menu/recipe
- Gathering necessary equipment and ingredients
- Following recipe or instructions
- Serving
- Eating
- Cleaning up
- Continuing to next activity

The activity lends itself to partial participation or collaboration since some components—especially serving and cleaning up—are substantial tasks in their own right.

The major decisions should address the range of items/menus to be prepared, and the format for presenting the target recipes or instructions. Picture recipes can be specific to each dish or designed to accommodate a range of items that require similar preparation.

ITEM 2-2-11   Preparing Meals
a. Breakfast	c. Dinner
b. Lunch	d. Snacks

Note: This activity can be coordinated with ITEM 2-2-10: Planning Meals, and ITEM 2-2-7: Buying Groceries. See Williams, J., & Horner, R. H. (1986). General case cooking. Unpublished manuscript, Specialized Training Program, University of Oregon, for a set of picture recipe cards designed to teach four general food preparation routines, each of which can be used with a large number of items.

There Is Always More Than One Way to Skin a Cat

. . . and more than one way to do most other activities as well. All we need to do is be creative.

If you identify an activity that you would like to target for your son or daughter or for a particular student or resident but it seems beyond his or her abilities, don't give up! Just think about it.

Look over the activity analysis to identify the steps of the activity that might present special problems. Then try to generate as many ways as possible that the step might be modified so that the individual can, indeed, complete the necessary performance aspects.

We know that this might be hard after years of hearing that your son or daughter didn't have the "prerequisite skills" or that the particular student "just wasn't ready" for the target activity. What we're telling you now is that one must modify the activity, not exclude the person with a disability because he or she can't do things "the normal way." For example, there are many ways to modify task performance for a person who is not skillful with money. Rather than expecting him or her to count out the exact amount of a purchase, one might arrange for him to pay with a $10 bill and simply hold his hand out for change (an "over-payment" strategy). Or one might teach her to count out the number of dollars indicated on the cash register display and then add one more (a "next-dollar" strategy). Or he or she might match real coins to coin stamp pictures that represent the target amount. Different strategies will be better for different activities and for different individuals.

There are a similar variety of ways to adapt tasks to accommodate people who have no reading skills, limited verbal language, or restricted motor abilities. There is always a way.

Space and Belongings

Supplies get used up. Things get broken. If life is to go on (and why shouldn't it?!), these items must be replaced.

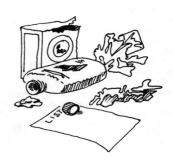

Activity includes:

- Determining target items
- Preparing to go (checking appearance; getting money, list, and other necessary materials)
- Traveling to store
- Entering
- Selecting target item(s)
- Paying for items
- Returning home
- Storing item(s) as appropriate
- Continuing to next activity

In most instances, it will be necessary to have a system for keeping track of supplies that need to be replenished. Logos, labels, empty containers, or shopping cards can be used to create a "list." A household should choose a strategy consistent with its meal-planning/grocery-shopping system.

There must be decisions regarding which stores will be patronized, and whether choice will be limited to specific brands and sizes. The payment strategy should be consistent with the adaptations made for other similar activities (such as purchasing groceries).

ITEM 2-3-1 **Purchasing Personal Items**
    a. Grooming supplies
    b. Household items/furnishings

When the going gets tough, the tough go shopping!!

Shopping for clothing items not only gets you out into the community, but also gives you an opportunity to make important choices about your wardrobe. Though it is hardly a daily activity, the need to purchase some type of garment is quite frequent.

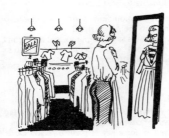

Activity includes:

- Deciding type of item to be purchased
- Preparing to go (checking appearance; getting money and other materials)
- Traveling to store
- Locating relevant department
- Locating items of correct size
- Selecting items and trying on if necessary/appropriate
- Paying for item
- Returning home/to next activity

Since the range of choice in this activity is so large, some limits will have to be defined in order to develop effective training. For example, it may be desirable to have the decision of what kind of item to buy (shirt, coat, underwear, etc.) made by the parent, an advocate, or a residential support person who is familiar with the person's wardrobe and clothing needs. Similarly, the general price range for the target garment may or may not be designated in advance. Shopping for all items will be facilitated if the shopper carries a card that lists his/her sizes for common items along with any preferred brand names.

ITEM 2-3-2 **Purchasing Clothing Items**

Unless you have a never-ending wardrobe, washing clothes is an inescapable fact of life.

Where and how you do it will, of course, depend on the resources in the home or neighborhood.

Using a regular machine includes:

- Gathering necessary supplies and materials (laundry, detergent, softener, etc.)
- Traveling to laundry area
- Loading clothes
- Adding detergent
- Setting temperature and cycle
- Activating machine
- Removing clothes at end of cycle
- Hanging clothes/putting clothes in dryer
- Returning supplies to storage
- Continuing to next activity

Using coin-operated equipment naturally adds expense . . . and several steps:

- Gathering necessary supplies and materials (laundry, detergent, softener, money, etc.)
- Traveling to laundry area
- Loading clothes
- Adding detergent
- Setting temperature and cycle
- Selecting coins
- Inserting coins
- Activating machine
- Removing clothes at end of cycle
- Hanging clothes/putting clothes in dryer
- Returning supplies to storage
- Continuing to next activity

Hand washing may be appropriate when very few or very delicate items need to be washed. This variation includes:

- Gathering necessary materials (laundry, special detergent)
- Traveling to sink or laundry room
- Filling sink
- Adding detergent
- Adding clothes
- Washing
- Rinsing items
- Wringing items dry
- Hanging clothes
- Returning supplies to storage
- Continuing to next activity

Hand washing will require a different type of detergent and sufficient space to hang items to dry.

The decision to wash all items in cold water eliminates the need to sort items by color and to choose among complex washer settings. Virtually everything can be washed successfully on a COLD setting.

Some detergents come in premeasured amounts (bags or tablets) or with built-in measuring devices (two pumps equals the necessary ¼ cup). Other products will require a strategy to assure that the necessary amount is measured (e.g., a measuring cup marked with a piece of tape at the appropriate volume).

Picture sequence cards can present information regarding the target temperature setting, the number and type of coins needed, and how to activate the machine.

Scheduling this activity at fixed intervals (e.g., every Sunday afternoon or every Thursday night) reduces the possibility of running short of clean clothes!

Many individuals will need assistance discriminating items that can be washed from those that must be dry cleaned (e.g., wool skirts or certain synthetic fabrics).

ITEM 2-3-3   Washing Clothes
a. **By regular machine**
b. **By coin-operated machine**
c. **By hand**

Note: This activity can easily be combined with ITEM 2-3-4: Drying Clothes and ITEM 2-3-5: Folding Clothes.

Drying clothes . . . with machines or with nature.

A simple but important contribution to the household . . . and your own closet.

With a *regular machine,* the activity includes:

- Gathering necessary materials (fabric softener sheets, hangers)
- Removing wet clothes from washer or basket
- Placing clothes and fabric softener sheet in dryer
- Setting temperature and drying time (if appropriate)
- Activating machine
- Removing clothes from dryer
- Hanging or putting away dry clothes
- Continuing to next activity

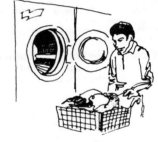

Using a *coin-operated* machine requires the additional steps of selecting and inserting coins.

The "low-tech" option requires sufficient space or line; and clothes pins, hangers, or some means of attaching clothes to the line.

Following this choice, the activity includes:

- Gathering necessary materials
- Attaching items to clothesline
- Removing items when dry
- Putting away dry clothes
- Continuing to next activity

ITEM 2-3-4   Drying Clothes
a. **Regular dryer**
b. **Coin-operated dryer**
c. **Line drying**

Note: This activity can be easily combined with ITEM 2-3-3: Washing Clothes and ITEM 2-3-5: Folding Clothes.

Something has to be done with those clothes once they are all dry!

A small but important task is to fold the clean laundry and return it to storage.

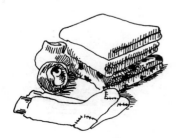

Activity includes:
- Removing laundry from dryer or clothesline
- Traveling to location with flat surface
- Pairing socks
- Folding or hanging items
- Grouping items by owner
- Returning items to target drawer/location
- Continuing to next activity

Picture sequence cards can be used to represent the pattern for folding various items. Garment labels can facilitate the sorting by owner. Alternately, the sorting can be handled by a second person or by having household members pick up their own folded clothes.

ITEM 2-3-5   Folding Clothes

Note: This activity is easily combined with ITEM 2-3-4: Drying Clothes.

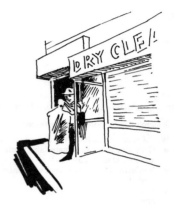

Wash and wear has almost *made ironing obsolete . . .*

. . .But there are still clothes that look better when they've been pressed.

Activity includes:
- Gathering necessary materials and equipment (board, iron, spray fabric sizing, hangers, etc.)
- Setting up ironing board
- Activating iron to desired temperature
- Ironing item(s)
- Folding item(s) or placing on a hanger
- Turning off and unplugging iron
- Returning equipment and material to storage
- Transferring clothes to closet/storage location

Specific components of the activity will differ depending on whether the board and iron remain set up in a permanent location (such as a basement or laundry room) or whether they are put up and taken down each time clothes are pressed.

ITEM 2-3-6   Ironing Clothes

Not a frequent event, but a "must" for some wardrobes.

Using the dry cleaners is an important errand in many households, and an activity one individual can perform for others. The activity actually includes two separate components: dropping things off and picking them up.

Dropping off cleaning includes:
- Preparing to go (collecting garments; checking appearance; getting money)
- Traveling to cleaners
- Entering

- Approaching counter
- Communicating name and instructions
- Taking claim check
- Returning home/to next activity

Picking up cleaning includes:
- Preparing to go (getting claim check and money, checking appearance)
- Traveling to cleaners
- Entering
- Presenting claim check/making request

- Paying
- Collecting cleaning
- Returning home/to next activity

The cost of the service will vary. Setting up an account at the cleaners will eliminate the need to pay for items directly. Communication cards—or standing instructions for garment care—can effectively meet communication demands of this activity.

Scheduling a regular day to perform this activity will help give it structure and allow for effective wardrobe planning.

ITEM 2-3-7   Using Dry Cleaner
   a.   Dropping off items
   b.   Picking up items

A never-ending task . . . almost.

Perhaps one of the most useful and appreciated activities an individual can do in his or her home is keep things tidy.

Activity includes:
- Traveling to target room
- Clearing objects from floor
- Removing objects from surfaces
- Returning items to designated locations
- Returning furniture/pillows/etc. to designated position
- Continuing to next activity

Designating particular room assignments and target times and/or days will enable this activity to be governed by an individual schedule.

ITEM 2-3-8   Straightening Up A Room
   a.   Bedroom   d.   Dining room
   b.   Living room   e.   Other
   c.   Basement

Note: This activity may be combined with ITEMS 2-3-15 through 2-3-18: Dusting, Sweeping, Vacuuming, or Mopping.

Though we live in a "throw-away society," in most households the dishes still need to get done . . . three times a day!

Doing dishes is an excellent way for youngsters to begin to take on "job responsibilities" at home and for adults to contribute to the maintenance of their household.

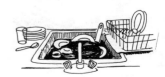

Activity includes:
- Rinsing dishes
- Preparing cleaning materials (filling the sink with water, scrubbers with soap, etc.)
- Cleaning the surfaces of each item

- Rinsing
- Placing dishes in drainer
- Cleaning up work area
- Continuing to next activity

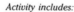

There are endless variations and adaptations to this task. For example, dishes can be washed in a sink that has been stopped and filled with water, in a dish pan, or even under running water with a soap-filled scrubber. A key to effective training is to determine a particular method. Each dictates a slightly different task sequence and demands slightly different motor responses. Dishes can be rinsed individually as they are put in a rack to dry or the entire rack can be rinsed with a hand held spray. The decision to clean dishes with a rag, a sponge, or a bristle brush has similar implications for training and performance.

Be clear about the materials and procedures that are to be used in this activity. Thoughtful decisions can eliminate the need to deal with complex discriminations. For example, if you have Teflon pans (or other with some "special" surface), all scrubbing tools should be "Teflon compatible" so that an individual does not have to make decisions about which tool to use for which dish and the probability of damaging pans is reduced.

Picture sequence cards can serve as a useful reminder of the critical steps of this activity and clearly define household standards.

Time required for this activity will depend on the number of dishes to be done.

This activity may present difficulties for individuals who have motor problems ... especially if dishware is breakable!

ITEM 2-3-9   Washing Dishes By Hand

Note: This activity can be combined with ITEM 2-3-12: Clearing the Table or ITEM 2-3-10: Drying Dishes by Hand.

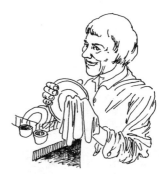

In some households, people dry dishes; in others, dishes dry themselves.

Drying dishes is a standard household chore and an easy way to make a contribution.

Activity includes:
- Getting dish towel
- Selecting an item
- Drying all surfaces of the item
- Replacing item in drawer/cupboard

- Cleaning up work area
- Returning towel to rack/hook
- Continuing to next activity

For someone who is short of stature, has limited strength or range of motion, or has difficulty classifying objects, the activity can be modified so that dried dishes are stacked on the counter and replaced in drawers/cupboards by another individual.

Time required for the activity will, of course, be a function of the number of dishes to be done!

ITEM 2-3-10   Drying Dishes By Hand

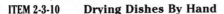

A dishwasher takes some—
but not all—of the work out of doing the dishes.

The question "Whose turn to *do* the dishes?" simply becomes "Who's going to *load* (or unload) the dishes?"

Loading the dishwasher includes:
- Rinsing food from dishes
- Placing items in correct position on rack

- Adding soap
- Activating machine
- Continuing to next activity

Unloading the dishwasher includes:
- Opening dishwasher
- Removing items to drawer or cupboard/counter

- Continuing to next activity

ITEM 2-3-11   Doing Dishes with the Dishwasher
     a. Loading the dishwasher
     b. Unloading the dishwasher

Clearing the table is a simple activity and one
that can be practiced and performed three times a day!

It is one of the first chores we all learn as we grow to be contributing members of our household. It is something we can do for ourselves or for others at mealtime.

Activity includes:
- Grasping item(s)
- Transferring item(s) from table to sink/counter

- Continuing to next activity

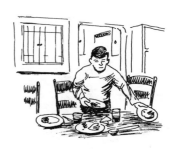

When the activity is done not only for oneself but for all people at a meal, additional elements include:
- Getting damp sponge or rag
- Clearing all items from table (placemats, condiments, etc.)
- Wiping table

- Replacing items
- Returning sponge/rag to storage
- Continuing to next activity

It is a household decision whether dishes should be transferred to the counter, sink, or directly into a dishwasher.

ITEM 2-3-12   Clearing the Table
     a. Own dishes
     b. All dishes

An activity for which there is ample opportunity for practice: Cleaning the kitchen.

The larger the household, the more often cleaning will be necessary. Though neither glamorous nor difficult, it's an activity much appreciated by housemates.

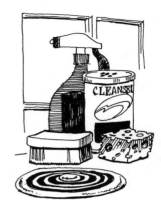

Activity includes:
- Gathering necessary supplies and materials (cleansers, disinfectant, sponges, etc.)
- Preparing cleanser as necessary
- Wiping entire surface
- Rinsing surface
- Returning materials to storage
- Continuing to next activity

It is important to specify clearly what "cleaning the kitchen" means: Counters? Sinks? Cabinet surfaces? Appliances? There may be slight variations in the materials used for each and, consequently, a need to develop a task analysis for individual components.

Picture cards are one way to specify what tasks are to be included, the order in which they are to be completed, and the particular cleaning products that are to be used.

Whether this activity is completed daily or weekly, it will help to have it scheduled on an individual's personal calendar!

ITEM 2-3-13   Cleaning the Kitchen

Note: This activity may be expanded to include sweeping or mopping kitchen floor or those activities may be selected independently and performed at separate times.

No home can afford a garbage strike!

Develop a contract now so that garbage is removed regularly.

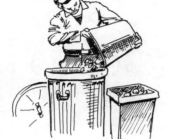

Activity includes:
- Traveling to trash can
- Removing trash bag/liner from can
- Fastening closure, if appropriate
- Depositing bag in garbage can or designated area
- Replacing trash bag/liner
- Continuing to next activity

Steps can be eliminated if garbage is dumped directly from one can into a larger can outside. Trash bags and liners, while clean and efficient, do add steps. And ties for some bags can be very perplexing, even for those of us with excellent fine motor skills.

The frequency with which the activity is performed will depend on the size of the household and the size of wastebaskets and garbage cans. Responsibility should be clearly noted on a personal schedule. A different schedule may be appropriate for kitchen garbage than for smaller wastebaskets throughout the house.

Picture cards may be needed as a "reminder" of the number and location of wastebaskets in the house.

ITEM 2-3-14   Taking Out the Garbage

Dusting . . . Dusting . . . Dusting . . . Dusting . . . Dusting . . . Dusting . . .Dusting

Necessary to maintain the appearance—and sanitation—of the household!

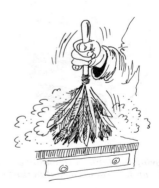

Activity includes:
- Gathering necessary materials (dustcloth, spray wax, etc.)
- Traveling to room
- Removing items from surfaces as necessary
- Dusting entire surface
- Replacing any objects on surface
- Completing each item/surface in room
- Returning materials to storage
- Continuing to next activity

There are a number of materials that can complicate the job and still others that can simplify the task. A variety of spray waxes add an extra step and require judgments about the duration—and direction!—of the spray. Feather dusters may be easier to grasp for some and do a good enough job to eliminate the need to move all items on a surface.

Picture cards can indicate items to be dusted and serve as the basis of a self-monitoring system to help the individual keep track of the job.

ITEM 2-3-15   Dusting

Your floors need it—every now and then.

And the larger and more active the household, it's more *now* than then.

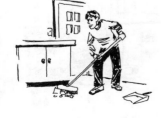

Activity includes:
- Gathering necessary materials (broom, dustpan)
- Traveling to room/area to be swept
- Sweeping surface area
- Disposing of debris
- Returning materials to storage
- Continuing to next activity

If the area to be swept opens to the outside, you may elect to sweep debris outside rather than into a dustpan.

Different surfaces (kitchen floor, living room, driveway) will require adjustments in the sweeping pattern used, and in the number and nature of obstacles that must be dealt with.

If more than one room/area is to be swept, consider a general case program to ensure ability to deal with variation in floor patterns.

ITEM 2-3-16   Sweeping

Rugs need cleaning, too.

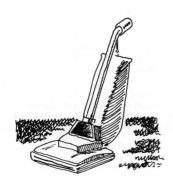

...and vacuuming sure beats beating the rugs!

Activity includes:
- Gathering necessary equipment (vacuum cleaner, extension cord, etc.)
- Traveling to target room
- Turning on vacuum cleaner
- Cleaning rugs/floors
- Turning off vacuum cleaner
- Returning equipment to storage
- Continuing to next activity

Variations in the activity will come as a function of the particular vacuum cleaner available. Machines differ in the on/off mechanism, whether various tools can be interchanged, settings for rug/floor type, and how/whether the cord retracts. Some machines may have the capacity to clean plain surfaces as well as rugs or carpet. Take care that individuals are able to use the particular equipment available in their own household.

Be sure to specify the room/areas for which the individual will be responsible. If there are many, it may be appropriate to build a general case program to deal with variation in furniture/floor plans.

ITEM 2-3-17　　**Vacuuming**
    a.　**Whole house**　　c.　**Bedroom**
    b.　**Living room**　　d.　**Other**

You can get down on your hands and knees but that's probably not necessary.

How much and how often you mop the floor depends on your home and your own standards for cleanliness.

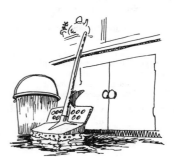

Activity includes:
- Gathering necessary materials (mop, bucket, cleanser, etc.)
- Filling bucket with water
- Adding cleanser
- Removing rugs, furniture, or other obstacles from surface
- Cleaning floor
- Disposing of water
- Returning materials to storage
- Continuing to next activity

Components of the activity may change as a function of the particular equipment and products used. Cleansers that are not diluted with water eliminate the need to measure water and detergent. The style of the mop itself will affect the particular motor requirements of the task. Picture self-monitoring cards can be used to sequence the steps of the activity, and a bucket and/or measuring cup can be modified with a piece of masking tape to take the guesswork out of how much water or cleanser to add.

Be sure to specify the rooms/areas for which the individual will be responsible.

ITEM 2-3-18　　**Mopping**
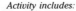
    a.　**Kitchen**　　c.　**Other**
    b.　**Bathroom**

Make yourself a hero at home: Clean the bathroom.

Typically, this activity is scheduled weekly but it may be necessary more often in large or busy households.

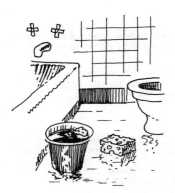

Activity includes:
- Gathering necessary tools and materials (cleansers, sponge, toilet bowl brush, etc.)
- Traveling to bathroom
- Removing rugs and articles from surfaces to be cleaned
- Cleaning bathtub
- Cleaning sink
- Cleaning toilet
- Cleaning mirror(s)
- Cleaning floors
- Returning materials to storage
- Continuing to next activity

Components of the activity will vary as a function of the particular materials and equipment used, and the bathroom fixtures and layout.

The activity can be completed by a single person or divided so that different people are responsible for different elements of the task in a "job-sharing" arrangement. Be sure to specify which elements are expected of each individual.

More detailed task analysis may be needed for each target element of this activity. Picture cards can be used to identify the particular materials/equipment needed and to define the particular task elements and the order in which they are to be completed.

In general, cleaning consists of: applying appropriate cleanser, rubbing the surface with a cloth/sponge/brush, and rinsing the surface with water. Storing materials in the bathroom itself will help streamline performance.

ITEM 2-3-19　　**Cleaning the Bathroom**

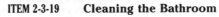

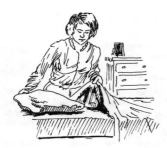

What a way to begin the day.

Making the bed gets you a good start on the day's business and helps make your bedroom a place you'd like to come home to.

Activity includes:
- Traveling to bedroom
- Removing pillow(s)
- Pulling up and straightening top sheet
- Pulling up and straightening blanket
- Adjusting spread/comforter
- Returning pillow(s) to bed
- Continuing to next activity

A number of decisions can significantly affect the complexity of this activity. Using a comforter permits much more flexibility and tolerance than does a bedspread. Similarly, a fitted bedspread provides built-in cues about what goes where and may be easier than other styles of spreads.

Making others' beds is also a way to contribute to general household maintenance.

ITEM 2-3-20   Making the Bed

Changing the bed reminds you that clean sheets are one of life's small pleasures.

Usually done once a week, this activity requires gross motor skills but few cognitive skills.

Stripping the bed includes:
- Removing spread/comforter and blankets
- Removing cover from pillow
- Removing top sheet
- Removing bottom sheet
- Taking used bed linen to laundry area
- Continuing to next activity

Making up the bed includes:
- Gathering clean sheets and pillow case
- Securing and smoothing bottom sheet
- Securing and smoothing top sheet
- Arranging blankets
- Arranging spread/comforter
- Covering pillow as necessary
- Continuing to next activity

The particular type of sheets and blankets will influence the complexity of this activity. Fitted sheets typically are easier to handle than those that require folded corners. Using an electric blanket will require additional components of plugging/unplugging blanket and arranging the control when stripping and making up the bed.

This activity can also be done for other members of the household.

ITEM 2-3-21   Changing Bed Linens
    a. Stripping the bed
    b. Making up the bed

Caring for a lawn or garden can be both work and recreation.

This activity offers a nice opportunity to enjoy the outdoors and contribute to household maintenance. And the list of chores is almost endless. Chores can be shared among household members or be the responsibility of a single "gardener."

It is important to designate which particular chores are expected. Picture cards can be used to define the expectations of each assigned task.

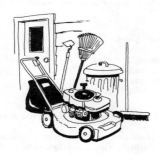

Watering can be done by hand or using a sprinkler. We favor using a sprinkler and an automatic timer. That variation of the activity includes:
- Attaching hose and sprinkler if necessary
- Setting sprinkler
- Turning on water
- Turning timer to designated time
- Continuing to next activity

If it is possible to leave the sprinkler and hose attached to the outside faucet, things are greatly simplified. Those who prefer the tidiness of hoses stored out of sight will have to add steps to the activity.

Raking can occupy nearly any weekend in the fall! The activity includes:
- Gathering necessary equipment (rake, trash bags)
- Raking leaves into piles
- Disposing of leaves (to compost, into trash bags, etc.)
- Returning equipment to storage
- Continuing to next activity

Mowing the lawn is a regular chore from spring through fall in most parts of the country and all year 'round in others. Though there will be some task variation as a function of the type of mower available, the general activity includes:
- Getting necessary equipment
- Turning on mower
- Mowing lawn area following designated pattern
- Turning off mower
- Returning equipment to storage
- Continuing to next activity

Training will be most effective if a clear decision is made about the particular pattern that will be followed (back and forth vs. perimeter vs. diagonal).

Weeding the lawn, flower beds, or garden is always a help. Training will require developing careful discriminations! *Activity includes:*

- Gathering necessary materials (knife, weeding fork, trash bag)
- Removing weeds from target area
- Disposing of weeds (into garbage bag)
- Returning materials to storage
- Continuing to next activity

Edging the lawn can be done with a gas or electric edger or with a muscle-powered version. The task varies considerably as a function of the equipment available. Using a power edger includes:

- Gathering necessary equipment (edger, extension cord, etc.)
- Turning on equipment
- Guiding edger along lawn borders
- Turning off equipment
- Returning materials to storage
- Continuing to next activity

Sweeping the porch/walk/driveway helps keep up appearances and cut down on the leaves and debris that are tracked into the house. *Activity includes:*

- Gathering necessary equipment
- Sweeping dirt/leaves/etc. toward collection point
- Disposing of dirt/leaves/etc.
- Returning equipment to storage
- Continuing to next activity

Variation in the style of broom (push broom vs. standard model) may affect performance of some individuals.

ITEM 2-3-22   **Doing Lawn Chores**

a.   **Watering**
b.   **Mowing the lawn**
c.   **Raking**
d.   **Weeding**
e.   **Edging**
f.   **Sweeping porch/walk/ driveway**

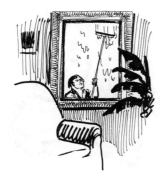

"But do they do windows?"

This standard inquiry of housekeepers attests to the importance of this activity—and to the general desire to have someone else do it!

Activity includes:

- Gathering necessary supplies and materials (window cleaner, paper towels, squeegee, etc.)
- Spraying on cleaner
- Wiping entire window area
- Returning materials to storage
- Continuing to next activity

There are many sources of task variation. Outside windows present slightly different demands than inside windows. Windows that must be removed from frames or combination windows where panels are raised and lowered are different from "plain" windows. Windows that require a ladder or step stool introduce still more modifications to the training analysis.

Even in the best of households, this is an infrequent, often seasonal activity. Consequently, it may be best to target the basic cleaning task and let variation be managed by a supervisor/ coworker.

ITEM 2-3-23   **Washing Windows**

Pets are good friends.

In fact, research shows that people with developmental disabilities who have pets are less likely to return to institutions than those who do not, and that elderly individuals who have pets to care for actually live longer. Pets help structure our day. They make us feel needed and loved.

There are many ways to help care for a pet, depending in part, of course, on the pet! And there is no limit on what can be a pet!

Feeding obviously is basic. *Activity includes:*

- Gathering necessary materials (food, dishes, can opener, etc.)
- Serving measured portion of food
- Returning material to storage
- Continuing to next activity

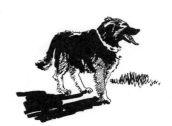

Picture sequence cards can be used to define any steps necessary to prepare the pet food (e.g., adding water or mixing dry and canned foods). Adaptations can be developed to ensure that the proper measure of food is presented.

Walking your dog is exercise for the two of you! *Activity includes:*

- Getting leash and other material (e.g., dog treats, pooper scooper)
- Attaching leash
- Walking
- Returning materials to storage
- Continuing to next activity

It may be important to have a carefully planned route that includes types of intersections that the individual can handle. Walking around the block, of course, eliminates the street-crossing problem without eliminating the exercise.

Grooming is something your pet will appreciate. *Activity includes:*

- Gathering necessary equipment (comb, brush, flea powder, etc.)
- Taking pet to designated area (porch, basement, or yard)
- Brushing or combing thoroughly
- Applying powder or other products as appropriate
- Returning materials to storage
- Continuing to next activity

Cleaning the cage for your pet is just as important as cleaning your own house. *Steps include:*

- Gathering necessary materials (garbage bag, newspaper, cedar shavings, gravel, etc.)
- Moving cage to an appropriate area for cleaning (basement, porch, etc.)
- Transferring pet to second container
- Removing used material
- Replacing gravel/bedding/paper
- Returning pet to cage
- Returning materials to storage
- Continuing to next activity

The precise steps of the task will, of course, depend on the particular materials contained in the pet's cage.

Cleaning the litter pan is a task that comes with a cat! *Task includes:*

- Gathering necessary materials (scoop, clean litter, detergent/spray disinfectant, etc.)
- Raking or dumping litter as per schedule
- Disposing of used litter
- Washing/disinfecting pan as per schedule
- Adding fresh litter to pan as per schedule
- Returning materials to storage
- Continuing to next activity

The schedule for this task will depend on the preference of the owner and the habits of the cat. Usually, fecal matter should be removed from the pan at least once a day and the litter changed and the pan cleaned once or twice a week.

It is important that all tasks associated with caring for a pet be included on the personal schedule or be publicly posted. The pet depends on us.

ITEM 2-3-24 **Caring for a Pet**

a. **Feeding**	d. **Cleaning cage**
b. **Walking**	e. **Cleaning litter pan**
c. **Grooming**	

If dog is man's best friend, surely plants are a close second!

Plants create a luxurious decor and provide the fun of watching something grow. Though they are not demanding, plants do require regular care.

Activity includes:

- Getting watering can (and any other materials)
- Filling can to designated level
- Watering plants
- Removing dead leaves/flowers
- Emptying can
- Returning materials to storage
- Continuing to next activity

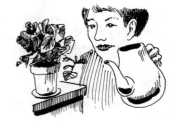

Photos may be used to indicate which plants are—or are *not*—to be included in the watering routine, and a weekly schedule can take the guesswork out of when to water.

A two-step process of pouring water into a measuring cup that holds the proper amount can ensure that plants get enough, but not too much water. There is, of course, less concern for detail when plants are hardy or when all can survive on a standard measure of water.

ITEM 2-3-25 **Caring for Plants**

Personal Business

Managing your own schedule is
perhaps the ultimate expectation of independence.

A personal schedule allows you to manage your time without necessarily having to tell time.

There are many ways to design a schedule to match the needs and skills of the user. A daily schedule can detail the morning routine, the schedule of tasks at work or school, and chores assigned at home. A weekly calendar can display appointments, special or nonrecurring tasks, or those activities scheduled less than once a week.

Individuals can assist in the selection and scheduling of leisure and personal management activities.

Schedules for home-based activities can be prepared weekly or adjusted each night for the following day. The schedule for work or school must, of course, be developed by people in those settings. Competent performance will be enhanced if a standard format is used across environments.

A picture of a clock face can designate *when* something is to be done and pictures or logos can replace written words to describe *what* should be done.

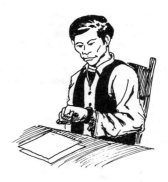

Activity includes:
- Locating personal schedule
- Matching time on clock to time on schedule
- Identifying activity associated with designated time
- Performing target activity
- Continuing to next activity

ITEM 2-4-1 Managing a Personal Schedule

Note: For procedures to teach self-monitoring, see Sprague, J., Mix, M., Wilcox, B., Styer, C., & Biber, E. (1983). Available from the Specialized Training Program, 135 College of Education, University of Oregon, Eugene, OR 97405.

Checks are both safer than cash and a necessity of modern life.

If you have an income or if you spend money, you probably need a checking account. Deciding where to bank is a matter of convenience and available services. The one-time-only task of opening an account is something that can be delegated to a family member/advocate.

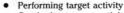

Making a deposit includes:
- Gathering necessary materials (checkbook, cash and/or check)
- Traveling to bank
- Completing deposit slip
- Endorsing check if necessary
- Submitting money/check to teller
- Balancing account
- Returning home/to next activity

Making a withdrawal includes:
- Gathering necessary materials (checkbook, purse/wallet)
- Traveling to bank
- Writing a check
- Submitting check to cashier
- Receiving money
- Balancing account
- Returning home/to next activity

Writing a check includes:
- Gathering necessary materials
- Filling out check
- Balancing account
- Continuing to next activity

Competence on this activity is increased if there is intensive discrimination training on whether a situation requires deposit or withdrawal or can be handled by writing a check.

Many adaptations of this activity are possible for students who lack the academic skills typically associated with banking. For example, an advocate can complete the check/deposit slip and the individual can either copy the information or can simply authorize the transaction. Individuals who cannot sign their name may use a sign or a name stamp. Balancing the account—which can be done by a friend or with the aid of a pocket calculator—can be completed at the time of the transaction or at some later time.

ITEM 2-4-2 Using a Checking Account
a. **Making deposits**
b. **Making withdrawals**
c. **Writing checks**

Maintaining a savings account is an
ideal way to prepare for a rainy day.

After some initial assistance in opening the account, the rest is easy.

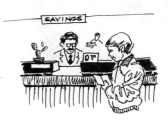

Making a deposit includes:
- Gathering necessary materials (bank book, money or check to be deposited, etc.)
- Traveling to bank
- Completing deposit slip
- Submitting deposit slip and money/check to teller
- Balancing account
- Continuing to next activity

Making a withdrawal includes similar steps. The only (!) difference is whether money goes in or comes out.

Since most financial establishments have separate slips for deposits and withdrawals, initial discrimination training may facilitate task performance.

There are several strategies that can support the participation of individuals without the normal repertoire of academic skills:

- Completing deposit/withdrawal tickets by matching-to-sample a form completed by a friend or advocate.
- Using a communication card to request that the teller complete the relevant deposit/withdrawal form.

- Balancing the account by using a pocket calculator.

ITEM 2-4-3   Using a Savings Account
    a. **Making deposits**
    b. **Making withdrawals**

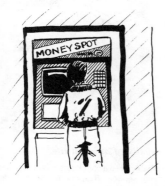

High tech comes to banking! Using a bank card enables you to withdraw money without having to write at all.

Depending on logistical considerations, using a cash card and conducting all transactions in cash may be more convenient than managing an account. However, don't think for a moment that using a cash card is necessarily easier than transactions involving a teller. Cash card use requires that the user discriminate the type of transaction, "remember" his or her access number, and be able to enter the correct amount of the transaction. And at some point, the account still must be balanced!

Activity includes:

- Preparing to go (gathering bank card and purse/wallet; checking appearance, etc.)
- Traveling to bank/cash machine
- Inserting card correctly
- Entering personal code

- Selecting transaction
- Entering amount
- Withdrawing money and card
- Replacing money, card, and receipt in purse/wallet
- Continuing to next activity

Using a cash card will vary somewhat as a function of the machine itself and the intended transaction. Since an individual typically will have accounts at a single bank, training should be designed to develop competence in responding to the single relevant machine.

ITEM 2-4-4   Using a Cash Card

Doctor. Case Manager. Dentist. Advocate.

Though we don't consult them daily, we do need them. And we need to know how to find them!

Using medical and social services includes behaviors as simple as travel from home or work to an appointment, and as complex as scheduling an appointment, keeping that appointment, and completing necessary forms.

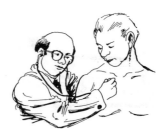

Procedures will differ for different service providers. Those with whom regular meetings are necessary (or advisable) will be the easiest to accommodate.

An individualized telephone directory is one adaptation to support such contacts. A personal weekly schedule that details appointments is also quite helpful.

Success in this activity will depend on clear decisions about which contacts and how much of the process the individual is to handle for himself or herself.

ITEM 2-4-5   Using Medical and Social Services

Note: Be sure to specify individual doctors or offices.

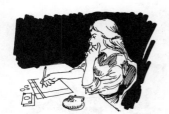

Budget balancing for the individual can be as complex as for the nation's treasury . . . and just as important!

There are of course numerous rules of thumb that can be used to guide the budgeting process, and there are some individuals with sufficient skills to "budget from scratch." For the majority of individuals with developmental disabilities, however, a budget will be something to be followed rather than developed. We recommend a process in which family and/or advocates review available income and expenses, and prepare a budget based on that information.

In general, it is wise for a budget to address only discretionary money; that is, only the amount available after the payment of rent and billed accounts. The target individual then learns to operate within that budget.

In one system, a standard amount is available for spending and that amount is divided into envelopes with a separate envelope for each day of the month. Unspent money from one day can be carried over to the next or deposited into a savings account.

In another system, discretionary income for a month is divided into four "weekly" envelopes. With this system, there is both greater choice and greater margin for error.

An alternative to budgeting is to have one's money parceled out into activity envelopes, each of which is identified by a picture/logo and contains enough money to purchase the designated activity.

ITEM 2-4-6   Budgeting Money

Something in life we can be sure of—bills!

And there is little choice but to pay them. The choice is merely whether to pay them in person or by mail. Paying in person has the advantage of maximizing visibility in the community but can be considerably more trouble than relying on the postal service. The decision is one that should consider an individual's present level of community integration and the logistics of travel.

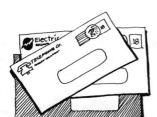

Paying by mail includes:
- Gathering necessary materials (statement, checkbook, stamps, envelopes, etc.)
- Completing check for target amount
- Inserting check and statement stub into envelope

- Addressing envelope
- Affixing stamp
- Mailing the letter
- Returning materials to storage
- Continuing to next activity

Paying in person includes:
- Gathering necessary materials (statement, checkbook)
- Completing check for target amount
- Preparing to go (checking appearance, gathering necessary materials)

- Traveling to business/designated location
- Submitting check with statement stub
- Continuing to next activity

For payment by check, an easy adaptation is to copy a sample check for the target amount. For payment in person, the check can be completed by one individual and carried to the business/service by another.

An individual might be responsible for all his/her bills, those of the entire household, or only a subset of a larger group.

ITEM 2-4-7   Paying Bills
a. By mail
b. In person

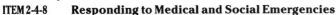

The best way to deal with an emergency is to prevent its occurrence!

Careful attention to the safety requirements of home and community activities is by far the most effective way of preventing emergencies.

By definition, an emergency is something out of the ordinary. While each will be unique—and not open to accurate "pretraining"—there are patterns of responding that can be applied across different types of emergency situations.

Selecting this objective as an IEP goal will require a careful decision about the particular strategy that will have most utility for the individual across the widest range of situations. Two of the most basic strategies are: seeking out a designated person or calling for help.

Either strategy requires significant initial support from a parent, teacher, or advocate to set up a functional system.

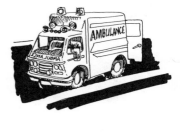

ITEM 2-4-8   Responding to Medical and Social Emergencies

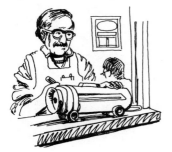

Shoes. Clothes. Hair dryers. Toasters. Cameras. Bicycles.

All of these things can wear out, tear, or break down.

Of course there will be variations in the activity as a function of the particular repair shop. Some items can be repaired while you wait, while others must be dropped off and picked up days later. Some services will require payment in advance while others will defer payment until the item is picked up.

Calling ahead to determine the procedures of the repair service and noting necessary pick-up dates on a personal schedule can help impose order on possible confusion.

Because this is a low-frequency activity, it may be most appropriate for individuals who already have a large repertoire of activities in the community.

ITEM 2-4-9   Purchasing Repair Services

Work

Introduction

Work is important. It is an expected part of an adult role in our society. It structures the day, provides access to a social network, and, perhaps most important, results in wages that can be used to create the kind of life-style we desire. It is through equal access to work opportunities that most minority groups have been able to enter the mainstream of society. The work component of a curriculum is central to achieving a quality adult life for individuals with disabilities.

Work is fundamentally different from the leisure and personal management domains. In both leisure and personal management, it is sufficient for a parent, advocate, or individual with a disability to select an activity for training or regular performance. Leisure activities that are available to citizens in a community are, by definition, available to young adults with severe handicaps. Most personal management activities are available to most individuals. It is the person with a disability (or family or advocates) who exercises the decision to include or not include an activity in the individualized plan.

In the work domain, by contrast, opportunities are not controlled by the decision of an individual with disabilities. Instead, opportunities depend on the willingness of employers and the success of social service programs in developing employment opportunities. While individual patrons decide whether to shop at a store, it is the store manager who determines who will *work* there.

Direct selection of a particular job is simply not possible, either for individuals with disabilities or for their nonhandicapped peers. Unemployment and underemployment are clear testimony to that fact. At the same time, however, there are more possible jobs or vocational training opportunities than any individual would ever select.

The challenge of the work domain is to make decisions that will maximize the probability of work and work-related benefits to individuals with disabilities. The choices individuals or their advocates are able to make are necessarily indirect.

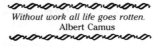

Without work all life goes rotten.
Albert Camus

Why Work?

Work is a means of generating wages and enjoying social integration. It is a medium for learning new skills, and expanding future choice. Finally, work-like activity is a way of keeping busy, staying visible in the community, and maintaining existing skills.

Work and work-related activity can serve several functions for an individual. Consider the activity "Cleaning a church." For one person, this "job" might be a volunteer activity done Saturday afternoons that allows the person to contribute to his or her congregation. Another individual might clean a church as a member of a janitorial training crew operated by the local community college. Still another individual might receive wages and ongoing support for cleaning a church twice weekly and maintaining its grounds.

An initial decision that parents and advocates must make in the individualized planning meeting is to establish the goal or purpose of work or work-related activity for the individual in question. Is the goal supported employment? Is it the development of work skills and, ultimately, greater vocational choice? Or is the goal informal preparation: being visible in the community, holding a part-time job, or making a contribution outside the home?

No other technique for the conduct of life attaches the individual so firmly to reality as laying emphasis on work; for his work at least gives him a secure place in a portion of reality, in the human community.
Sigmund Freud

How this Section of *The Activities Catalog* is Organized

Material in the work domain is divided into eight "job clusters," or different kinds of work an individual might perform. Within each job cluster are examples of things a person might do if the purpose of work were supported employment, if it were training, and if it were informal training/keeping visible.

The illustrations should serve a brainstorming function to help the catalog user identify similar opportunities that may be available or could be developed in his or her community. The examples represent the types of tasks and businesses where individuals with severe disabilities have been employed, received training, or worked as volunteers.

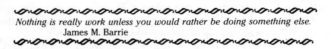

Nothing is really work unless you would rather be doing something else.
James M. Barrie

How to "Place an Order" for Activities in the Work Domain

1. *Determine the purpose of work for the target individual.* Be clear about the intended benefits. For high school students, the purpose will most often be training: developing work skills and expanding options to enhance choice. Informal or home-based work activities may also be appropriate if part-time jobs are available or if regular community service is a central part of the life-style of the family or household.

   For individuals who have graduated from school and for whom no services are available—who languish on human service waiting lists until funds for service expansion are available—the likely goal will be some sort of informal, home-based work activity. In the absence of services, parents and advocates seek strategies that will maintain the individual's profile with potential employers, maintain existing skills, and ensure that time is occupied with constructive activity.

   For individuals in service programs or in transition from school when employment services are available, the clear goal is supported employment. Supported employment is a recent federal initiative that stresses the importance of paid employment and of work in integrated worksites for individuals with the most severe disabilities. Supported employment emphasizes "support in employment" rather than an endless "preparation for employment." (For further information on supported employment, see Bellamy, G. T., Rhodes, L. E., Mank, D. M., & Albin, J. M., [in press]. *Supported employment: A community implementation guide.* Baltimore: Paul H. Brookes Publishing Co.)

2. *Decide the kind of work an individual will do.* In essence, select a job cluster. This decision can be based on performance in previous jobs or training situations, on what the person tells you, on general information about the person, or on the general demands of a particular kind of work.

3. *Select a training format.* In essence, this is a decision about the level of supervision the individual will need on the job. An individual job? Support within an enclave? Participation on a crew?

4. *Go for it!* Find or develop training and placement opportunities that meet individual needs. Or advocate that such opportunities be developed by schools or postschool providers. For volunteer placements, the hustle will have to be all yours!

Which of us . . . is to do the hard and dirty work for the rest—and for what pay? Who is to do the pleasant and clean work, and for what pay?
John Ruskin

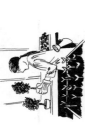

3-1   Agriculture and Natural Resources

This job cluster includes activities concerned with propagating, growing, caring for, and gathering plant and animal life and products. It also includes caring for plants, gardens, and grounds.

Purpose	Format	Tasks	Location
Supported Employment (Wages and Integration)	Individual Job	Sweeping cages Filling automatic feeders	Municipal Zoo Yelson's Egg Farm
	Crew	Mending fences Groundskeeping Cleaning stables Roadside cleanup	Area ranches City Parks and Recreation Department Arlington Racetrack County Maintenance Division
	Enclave	Raising seedlings	Greenthumb
Training (Skill Development and Choice)	Individual Job	Watering and repotting plants Cleaning cages	Woodruff's Nursery County Animal Shelter
	Crew	Maintaining lawns and practice fields	Central High School
	Enclave	Grading and boxing produce	University Orchards
	Other	Completing projects in horticulture class	Thurston High School
Informal Training or Volunteering (Visibility)	Individual Job	Gathering eggs Weeding the yard Cutting the grass Walking dogs Grooming horses	Neighbors' farms Home Home and neighbors' lawns Area dog owners Farm of relative
	Crew	Laying irrigation tiles Harvesting produce	Family farm Area orchards and fields
	Enclave		

51

3-2 Distribution

This job cluster includes any activities concerned with handling, processing, or retailing materials. Machinery may be involved in handling or processing operations.

Purpose	Format	Tasks	Location
Supported Employment (Wages and Integration)	Individual Job	Working as a baker's helper	SunRise (a cooperative bakery run by six employees with developmental disabilities and six people without disabilities)
		Loading goods	House of LaRose Beverage Distributorship
		Bagging garments	Aaron's Bulk Dry Cleaners
	Crew	Stocking shelves	Good Warehouse
		Sorting paper products	Northwest Re-Cycle (an enterprise that recycles paper products)
	Enclave	Silk screening t-shirts	Metrographics
Training (Skill Development and Choice)	Individual Job	Working as an audiovisual assistant	Queen Anne High School
		Collecting attendance slips	Lake Stevens High School
		Sorting bottles and cans for recycling	Albertson's Grocery
		Boxing chocolates	Euphoria Chocolate Company
		Pricing items	K-Mart
		Restocking vending machines	McMinnville Community Center
	Crew	Stocking and facing shelves	Rayson's 24 Hour IGA
		Pricing items	BiMart Discount Store
	Enclave	Labeling and filing films	Educational Resource Center
	Other	Attending a vocational education class	South Burlington High School

Informal Training or Volunteering (Visibility)		
Individual Job	Selling cards/magazine subscriptions Taking tickets Handling a paper route	Neighborhood Emerald Stadium Neighborhood
Crew	Canvassing for a political candidate Distributing literature for a bond issue Boxing food	Flexible; assigned by campaign manager Neighborhood First Hill Food Bank
Enclave		

I'm a great believer in luck, and I find the harder I work the more I have of it.   Thomas Jefferson

3-3 Domestic and Building Services

This job cluster includes activities concerned with providing domestic services to private households or lodging establishments, maintaining and cleaning linens/apparel in a commercial establishment, and performing cleaning or maintenance services to the interiors of buildings.

Purpose	Format	Tasks	Location
Supported Employment (Wages and Integration)	Individual Job	Cleaning restrooms Working as a housekeeper's assistant	County government complex Good Shepherd Retirement Center
	Crew	Dumping trash cans and dusting Cleaning tubs and sinks Picking up litter and sweeping sidewalks Cleaning houses	Insilco Center Building Howard Johnson's Motor Lodge Summit Mall Dust Busters (a cleaning service that employs individuals with and without disabilities)
	Enclave	Running washer and dryer, folding linens, and stacking delivery carts	Laundry Room, Eugene Hospital and Clinic
Training (Skill Development and Choice)	Individual Job	Cleaning glassware Washing, drying, folding, and restacking towels	Biology and Chemistry Departments, South Eugene High School Far West Fitness Club
	Crew	Cleaning out washers and dryers Emptying trash cans and ashtrays Cleaning seats, seat backs, and floors	Seawest Coin Operated Laundry Valley River Center Shopping Mall Cinerama (a four-theatre complex in a shopping mall)
	Enclave	Changing linens, dusting, vacuuming, and cleaning a block of four guest rooms	Sunset Motel
	Other	Completing tasks in a "domestic services training program"	Evergreen Community College

Informal Training or Volunteering (Visibility)	Individual Job	Cleaning house	Home of invalid neighbor
	Crew	Cleaning sanctuary, chapel, and classrooms	Westminster Church
	Enclave		

Anyone can do any amount of work provided it isn't the work he is supposed to be doing at that moment.
Robert Benchley

Training and Support Formats

There are, of course, many ways to provide training to individuals with severe disabilities while they are in high school and to support them in work placements after they have "graduated."

Having available an array of individual jobs, crews, and enclaves in a community increases the probability that adolescents and adults with severe handicaps will have an opportunity that matches their needs.

An *individual supported job* is a work station in the public or private sector in a service or industrial setting designed to accommodate a single employee or student. Supervision and training is initially provided by school staff or by employment program personnel who have completed a comprehensive job analysis. Performance is maintained through contact with indigenous supervisors and co-workers, with ongoing support from school or program staff. Individual job sites may be developed in any job or job cluster.

A *mobile work crew* is an instructional and organizational format designed to train or employ three to five individuals. The crew performs similar jobs in several different settings. Supervision, training, and ongoing support are provided by school personnel or a crew leader employed by the service program. Crews may be utilized in any job or job cluster that allows efficient division of job requirements into functional work tasks. Crews can operate quite well in service or industrial settings in public or private sectors. A single crew can accommodate individuals with a wide range of functioning levels.

An *enclave* is a format designed to provide employment or training to up to eight individuals in a single public or private sector service or industrial setting. Supervision, training, and ongoing support is provided by school personnel, by staff from an employment program, or by line supervisors within the business itself. Individuals may work in a specially supervised group within the setting or be distributed to work stations in various parts of the business. Job assignment and design is based on a comprehensive analysis of all jobs in the worksite.

An enclave may be utilized in any job or job cluster that allows efficient division of job requirements into functional work tasks.

Whether there is an enclave or a crew or individual supported jobs in any particular community business will depend on the size of the business, the type of work done, and the preferences of the management.

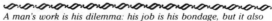

A man's work is his dilemma: his job is his bondage, but it also gives him a fair share of his identity and keeps him from being a bystander in somebody else's world.
Melvin Maddocks

3-4   Food Preparation and Services

This job cluster includes activities concerned with preparing food and beverages and serving them to patrons of such establishments as hotels, clubs, and restaurants. It also includes activities that maintain kitchen work areas and equipment or that maintain customer eating areas.

Purpose	Format	Tasks	Location
Supported Employment (Wages and Integration)	Individual Job	Cooking and bagging french fries Busing tables Washing pots Setting up and maintaining salad bar	McDonald's Restaurant Greentree Restaurant Ramada Inn King's Table Restaurant
	Crew	Delivering meal trays	Pacific Childrens' Hospital
	Enclave	Packaging silverware and condiments	Midwest Air Catering Service
Training (Skill Development and Choice)	Individual Jobs	Loading, running, and unloading dishwasher	Granite High School Cafeteria
	Crew	Setting and busing tables	Doctors' Lunch Room at McKenzie Willamette Hospital
	Enclave		
	Other	Participating in food services training program	Mt. Hood Community College
Informal Training or Volunteering (Visibility)	Individual Job	Cleaning up kitchen Preparing ingredients for chili for Sierra Club fund raiser Operating pop dispenser	Valley View Nursing Home Kitchen in area church Concession stand at school dance
	Crew	Delivering meals to individuals who are elderly "shut-ins" Preparing burritos	Meals-on-Wheels Rita's Burritos food booth at Saturday Market
	Enclave		

57

3-5 Office and Business Services

This job cluster includes activities concerned with recording, transcribing, reproducing, organizing, and distributing data, records, and communications. It also includes activities related to receiving, storing, and shipping goods and materials from an office/business.

Purpose	Format	Tasks	Location
Supported Employment (Wages and Integration)	Individual Job	Carrying inter-office memos Operating electric collator Running postage machine Entering data on traffic offenders into central computer	International Building at Data Corp Campus Press, State College Mail room of Donald Steld & Associates City Court office
	Crew	Preparing bulk mailing	Pacific Utility Company
	Enclave	Working in receiving division preparing new arrivals Microfilming canceled checks	University library First Interstate Bank
Training (Skill Development and Choice)	Individual Jobs	Running a copy machine Working as a library aide (clearing tables, reshelving books) Working as a receptionist Entering attendance data into computer	Oregon Research Institute Forest Grove High School School District Offices Woodburn High School Attendance Office
	Crew	Folding, stapling, affixing postage and mailing labels for monthly district-wide newsletters	School District Central Office
	Enclave	Microfilming records	Minuteman Insurance Group
	Other	Completing projects in an office skills training program	North Eugene High School

Informal Training or Volunteering (Visibility)	Individual Job	Folding and addressing weekly bulletins	Westmoreland Church
	Crew	Preparing mailings	Red Cross Central Office
	Enclave		

Who first invented work, and bound the free
And holiday-rejoicing spirit down?
Charles Lamb

3-6   Construction

This job cluster includes any activities concerned with fabricating, erecting, installing, paving, painting, and repairing structures such as buildings or roads.

Purpose	Format	Tasks	Location
Supported Employment (Wages and Integration)	Individual Job	Working as a painter's helper Running a planer	Yesterday's Dream (a small company focusing on building restoration) Homes Plus (a company specializing in pre-fabricated housing)
	Crew	Holding signs for a road crew	Variable
	Enclave	Fabricating stamped concrete sections	The Cement Works
Training (Skill Development and Choice)	Individual Job	Working as a carpenter's helper	Woodmasters
	Crew	Working to clean up area construction sites	Cascade Construction Company
	Enclave	Attaching hardware to cabinets	Pacific Cabinetmakers
	Other	Completing projects in a woodshop class	Hazen High School
Informal Training or Volunteering (Visibility)	Individual Job	Painting fences Removing old wallpaper to prepare wall for painting	Grandparents' farm Home of family friend
	Crew	Assisting father and neighbor build a deck	Home
	Enclave		

Wages versus Volunteering

The question of wages for workers with severe handicaps is one that has sparked recent controversy. Some have suggested that social interaction is so important that volunteering in a community site is more important than being paid for the work. The choice is a false one: it is clear that wages and social integration are not mutually exclusive. The federal government's supported employment initiative stresses the importance of both.

It is our strong feeling that people with severe handicaps should volunteer for the same reasons and in the same type of situations as do people without apparent handicaps. People may volunteer to support a cause. They may volunteer when they have no need for money, when they have no interest in regular employment, or when they need an activity to help structure their time. Still others may volunteer as a strategy to gain experience or to increase their visibility with the hope of eventual paid employment where they volunteer.

Just as these are valid reasons for people without disabilities, so do they justify nonpaid work by individuals with severe handicaps. The litmus test for volunteering by an individual with developmental disabilities is whether or not there are people without handicaps in similar volunteer roles.

It is also our strong feeling that people with severe handicaps should be paid for their work. Wages are perhaps the most significant benefit of work. It is in part through our salary that we judge our success, and wages allow us access to a wide range of other opportunities. For individuals whose productivity does not meet minimum wage standards, there are waivers that permit payment based on the level of productivity.

For further information about rules governing volunteering and about payment of subminimum wage, contact your regional office of the U.S. Department of Labor.

"A fair day's wages for a fair day's work": it is as just a demand as governed men ever made of governing. It is the everlasting right of man.
Thomas Carlyle

Time Devoted to Work

Time is an important dimension of any activity. In the work domain, time is especially important. While individuals are in high school, parents, teachers, and advocates must make decisions about how much of the school day should be devoted to work training.

After graduation, they may have to decide whether part-time work is acceptable. The latter decision will depend on the benefits of the job, and the life-style of the individual's household. In many cases, a part-time job will provide higher wages and greater social integration than will placement in a traditional day or work activity program. At the same time, however, part-time work may present significant management problems (e.g., What will the individual do the other 4 hours each day?)

While individuals with severe handicaps are still in school, it is considerably easier to offer a rule to govern the amount of time allocated to work training: as the student gets older, the amount of time spent should increase accordingly. Younger students might spend a minimum of 5 hours per week on job training in the community, while older students might spend virtually their entire school week at a job site.

Because of the learning characteristics of individuals with severe handicaps, it is important that there be ample opportunities to practice work skills. Thus, rather than work 5 hours, 1 day a week, it would be more appropriate to work 1 hour a day, five days a week.

An individual may, of course, receive training simultaneously on more than one job, but the training schedule for each job should allow ample opportunity for practice (e.g., at least 1 hour a day).

3-7   Health Occupations

This job cluster includes any activities concerned with maintaining the health, comfort, or safety of individuals. Also includes activities that involve the handling of medicine or materials that are used in hospital care.

Purpose	Format	Tasks	Location
Supported Employment (Wages and Integration)	Individual Job	Sterilizing medical instruments Operating the centrifuge	Carle Clinic Eastlake Medical Laboratories
	Crew	Assembling sterile packs for the Delivery Room	Central Metropolitan Hospital
	Enclave	Repackaging medical supplies	Supply room at Park Valley Hospital
Training (Skill Development and Choice)	Individual Job	Working as a child-care helper (washing toys, serving snacks) Working in nurse's office	Pee Wee Day Care Center Shelton High School
	Crew	Changing bed linen	Mercy Hospital
	Enclave		
	Other	Completing tasks delineated in a nurse's aide training program	Renton Vocational Technical Institute
Informal Training or Volunteering (Visibility)	Individual Job	Working as a candy striper Volunteering as a "companion" Babysitting	Burnham City Hospital Mt. View Care Center Homes in neighborhood
	Crew		
	Enclave		

3-8 Manufacturing and Machine Operations

This job cluster includes activities concerned with using tools and machines to fabricate, inspect, or repair products.

Purpose	Format	Tasks	Location
Supported Employment (Wages and Integration)	Individual Job	Using a multi-meter to test cable assemblies for microcomputers Working in a plywood mill	Spectra Physics Cornwall Lumber Company
	Crew	Building pallets	Rainier Pallet Corporation
	Enclave	Working as an electronics assembler in components for biomedical equipment	Physio Control Corporation
Training (Skill Development and Choice)	Individual Job	Operating a planer Using a heat sealer to repackage plumbing supplies for retail sales Hand soldering circuit board components	Seneca Sawmill Delta Fixtures Olympic Electronics
	Crew		
	Enclave		
	Other	Completing projects in a basic electronics class	Aberdeen High School
Informal Training or Volunteering (Visibility)	Individual Job		
	Crew	Building birdhouses for sale at church bazaars	Home
	Enclave		

63

There is no substitute for hard work.
Thomas A. Edison

3-9   Miscellaneous Occupations

This cluster includes a variety of activities that fall outside the job clusters previously described.

Purpose	Format	Tasks	Location
Supported Employment (Wages and Integration)	Individual Job	Working as a beautician's assistant (sweeping up hair, sterilizing combs and brushes, washing curlers)	Hair Masters Salon
	Crew	Working as a mover's helper / Detailing buses	Zimmerman Moving and Storage / Metro Transit Authority
	Enclave		
Training (Skill Development and Choice)	Individual Job	Washing cars / Working as a locker room attendant	Used Car Division, Williams Pontiac Dealership / Firestone High School
	Crew	Detailing school buses	School District Bus Barn
	Enclave		
	Other	Completing activities of a basic automotive shop class	Florence High School
Informal Training or Volunteering (Visibility)	Individual Job	Working as an usher	Beacon Hill Church
	Crew	Working at a car wash fund raiser for Cystic Fibrosis	Ray's Texaco Station
	Enclave		

64

Activities Pictures

The following pages contain pictures of 112 leisure, personal management, and work activities described in this catalog. These pictures may be reproduced, mounted on heavy paper or cardboard, and then used to help the individual select and order a variety of activities.

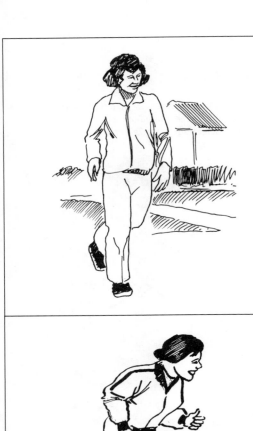

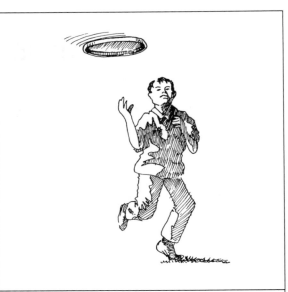

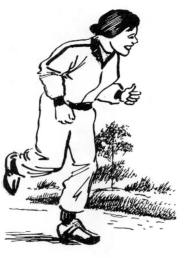

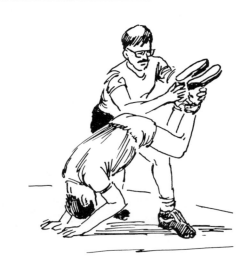

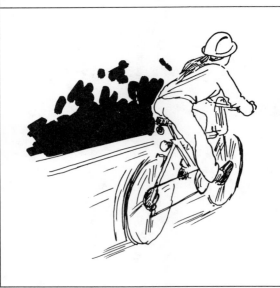

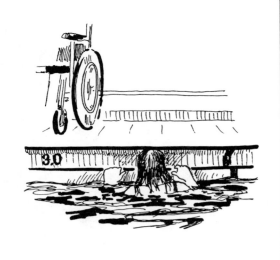

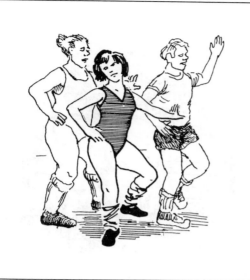 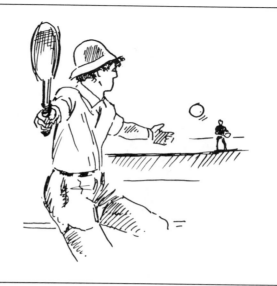

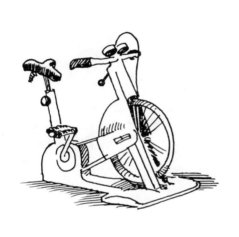 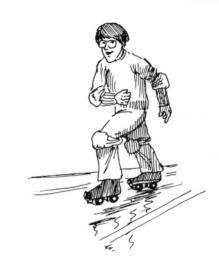

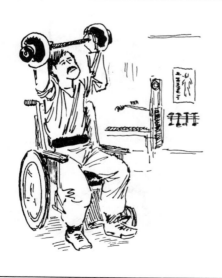 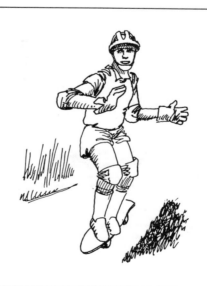

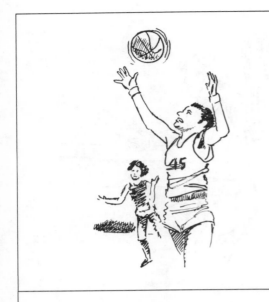
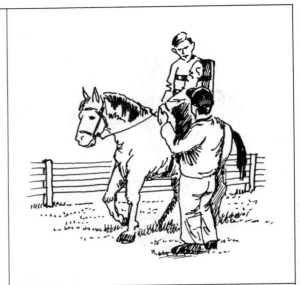
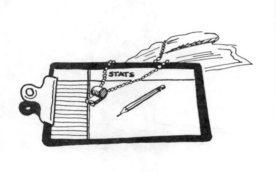
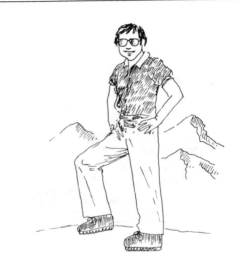
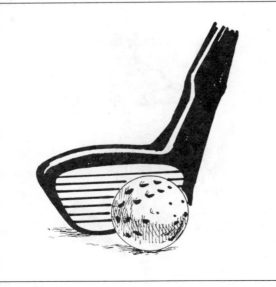
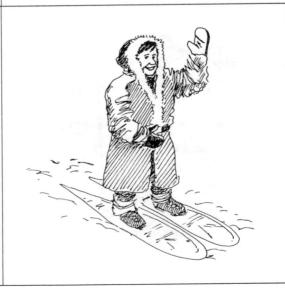

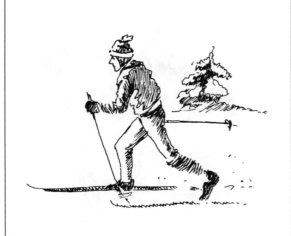

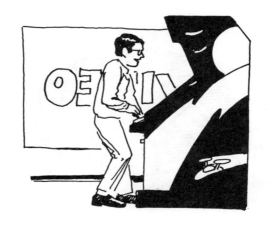

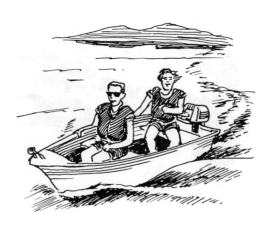

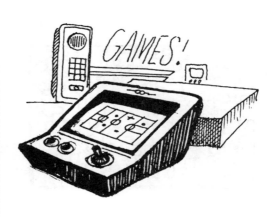

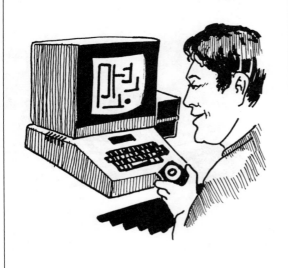

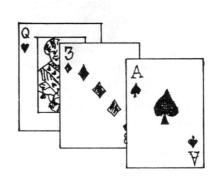

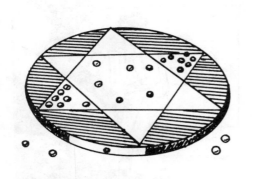

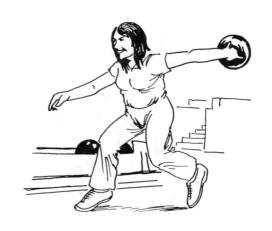

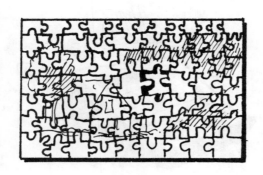

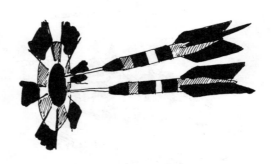

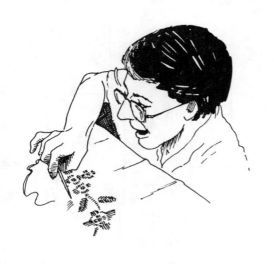

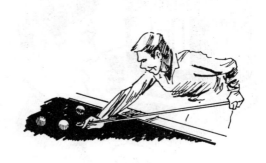

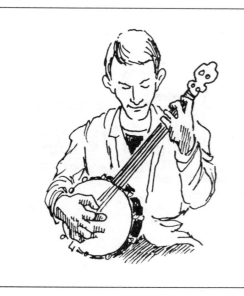

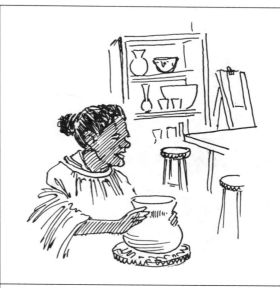

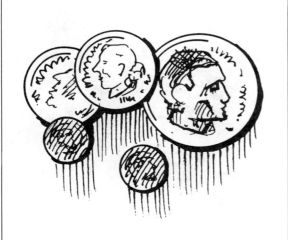

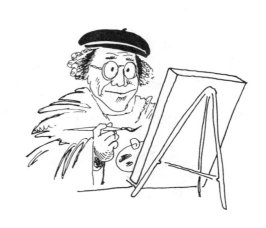

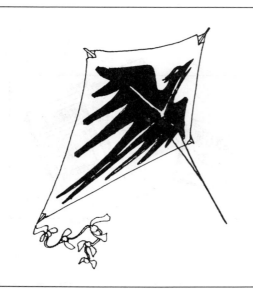

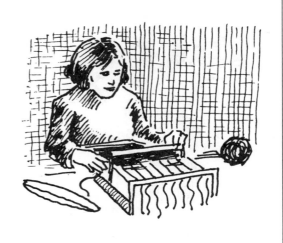

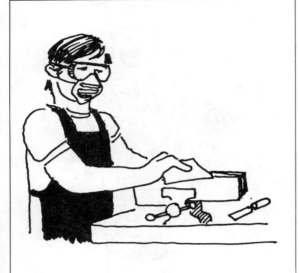

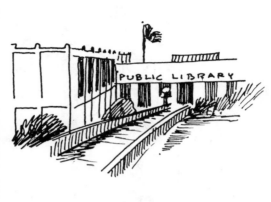

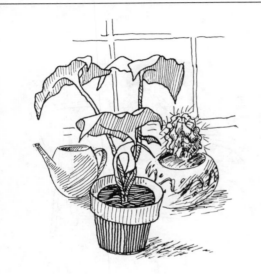

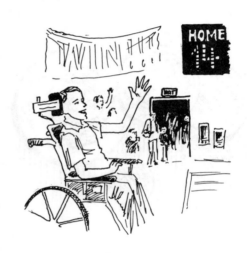

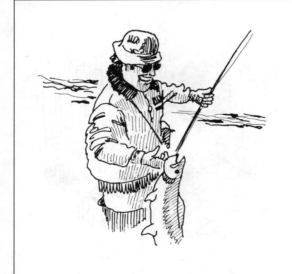

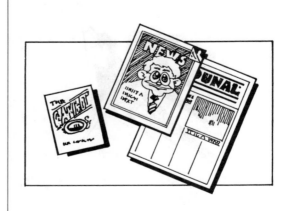

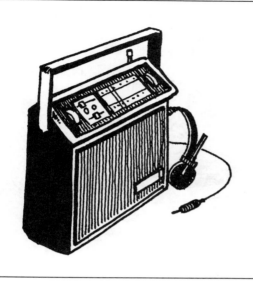

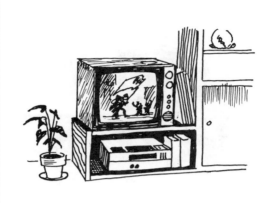

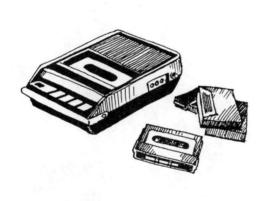

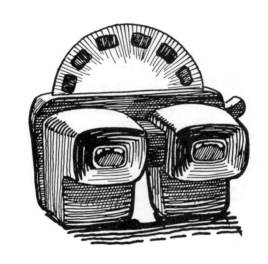

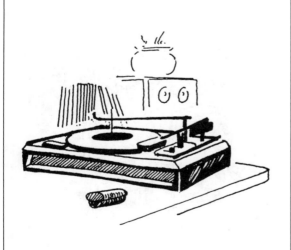

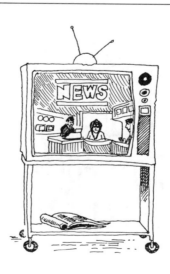

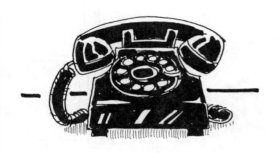

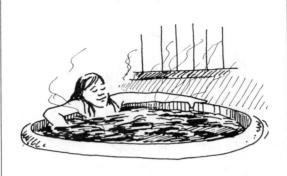

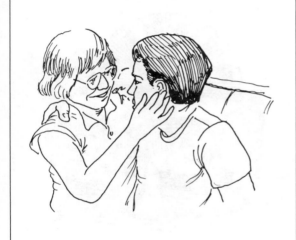

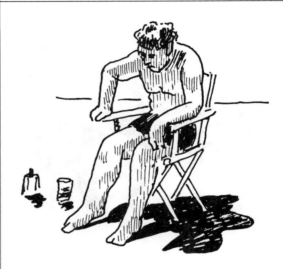

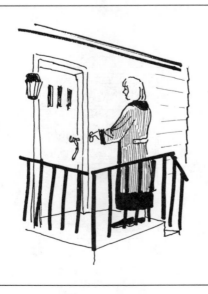

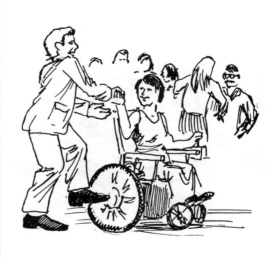

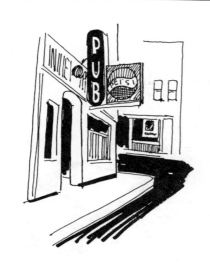

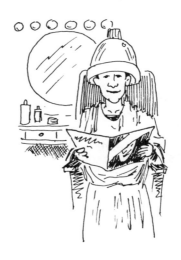

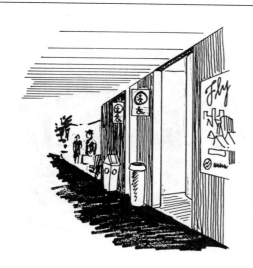

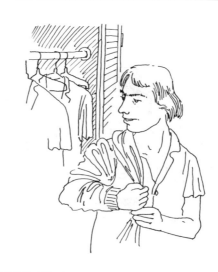

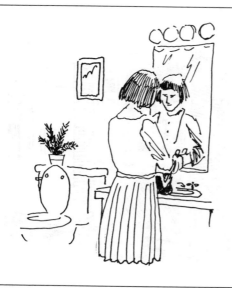

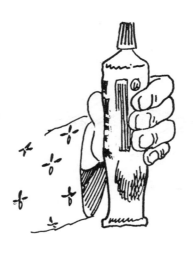

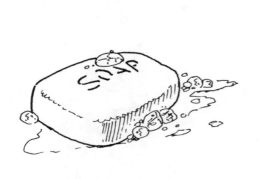

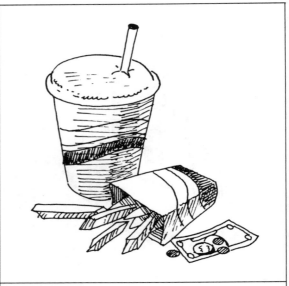

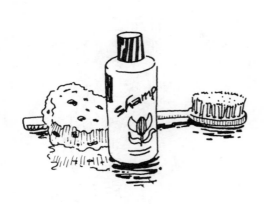

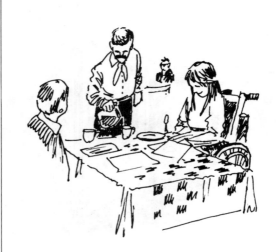

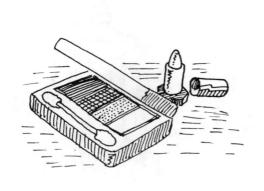

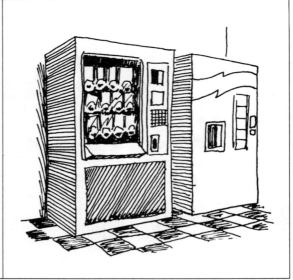

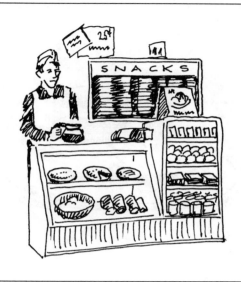

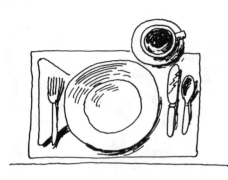

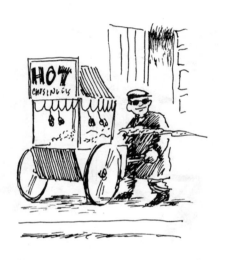

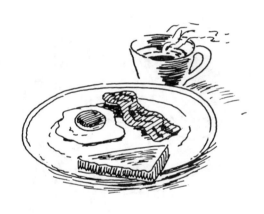

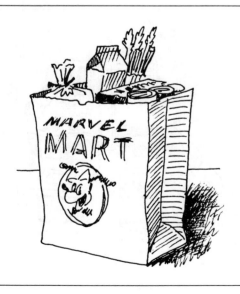

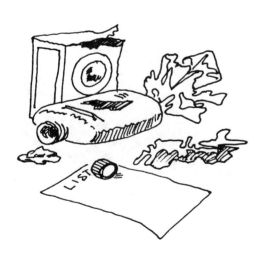

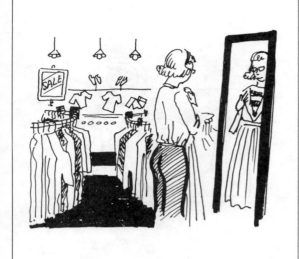

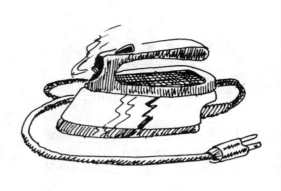

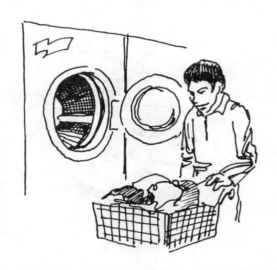

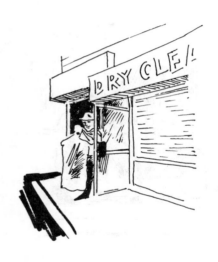

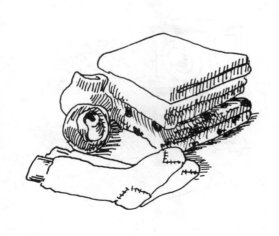

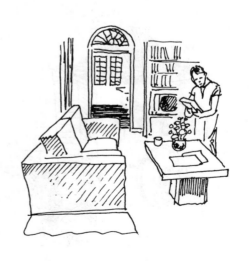

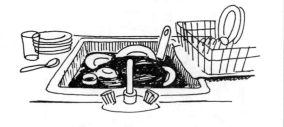

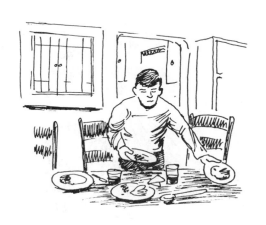

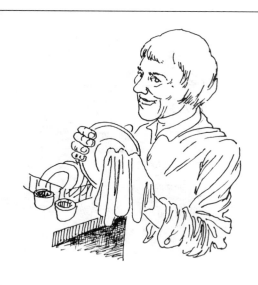

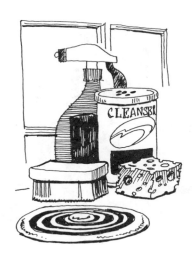

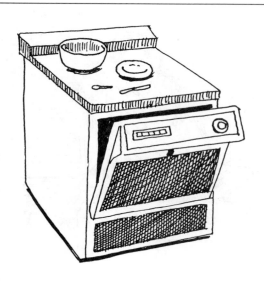

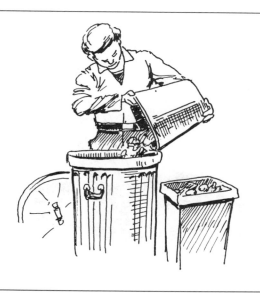

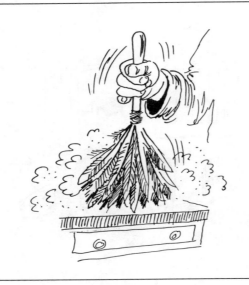

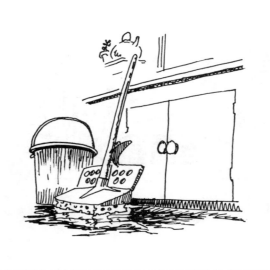

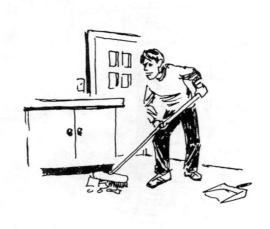

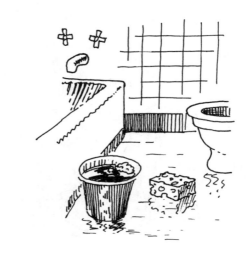

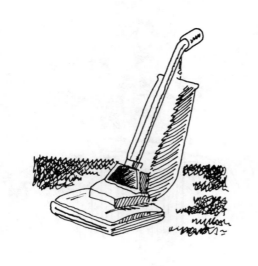

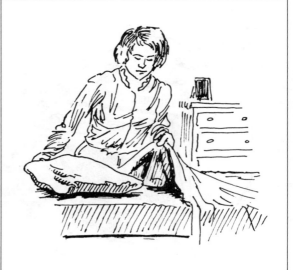

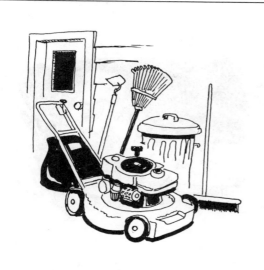

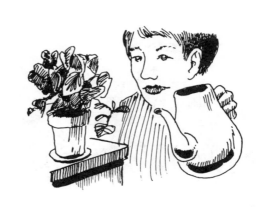

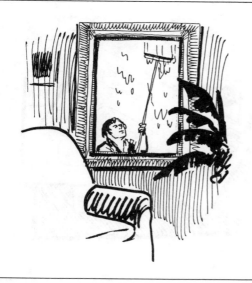

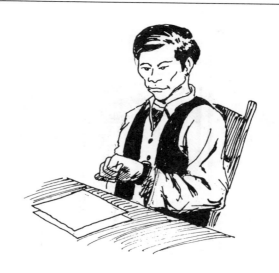

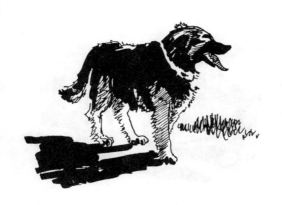

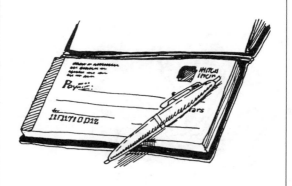

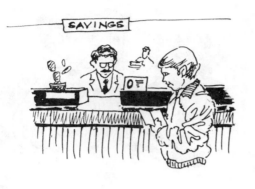

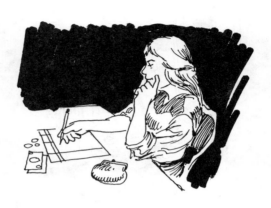

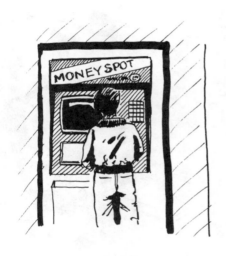

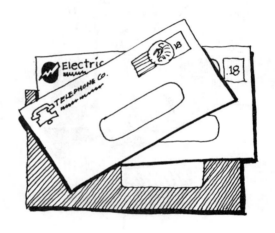

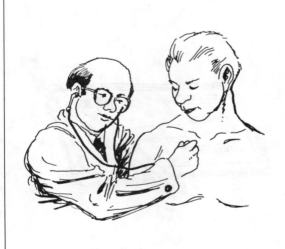

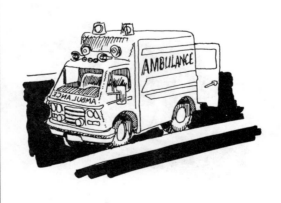

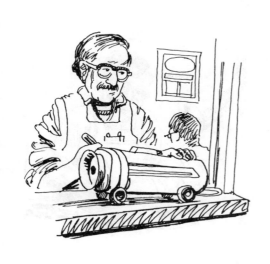

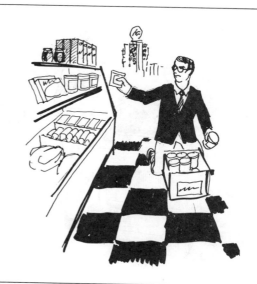

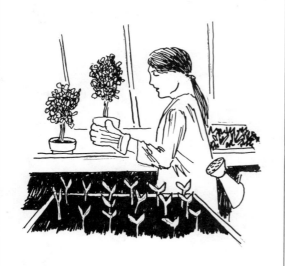

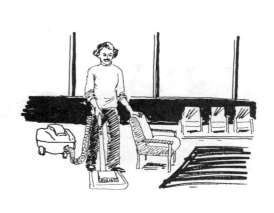

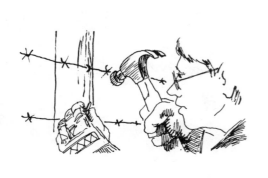

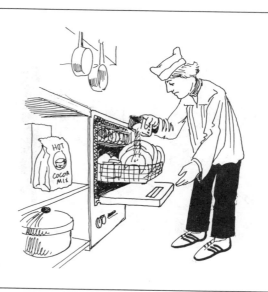

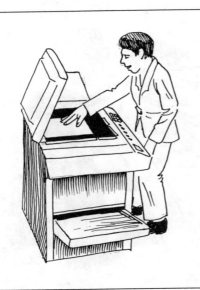

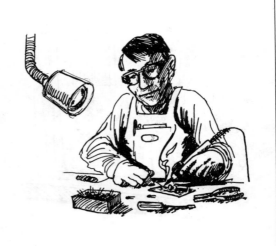

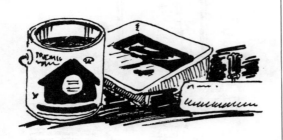

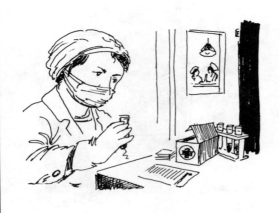

Activity Order Form

Leisure Domain
1-1 Exercise
1-2 Games/Crafts/Hobbies
1-3 Events
1-4 Media
1-5 Other

		Items Ordered	
Category	Item Number	Activity Description	Comments

Choose some items from each category. It is good to have a balance between things to do alone and things to do with others. It is also good to choose some activities that are constantly available and some that follow a schedule.

For office use only	
Total Items	
Total Categories Sampled	

Personal Management Domain
2-1 Self
2-2 Food
2-3 Space and Belongings
2-4 Personal Business

		Items Ordered	
Category	Item Number	Activity Description	Comments

Choose activities from all categories. Select items that are important for the household.

For office use only	
Total Items	
Total Categories Sampled	

Work Domain
3-1 Agriculture and Natural Resources
3-2 Distribution
3-3 Domestic and Building Services
3-4 Food Preparation and Services
3-5 Office and Business Services
3-6 Construction
3-7 Health Occupations
3-8 Manufacturing and Machine Operations
3-9 Miscellaneous Occupations

	Items Ordered	
Job Cluster	Support or Training Format	Comments

Possible support or training formats include Individual job, Crew or Enclave. Comments should include hours, possible tasks and location. Note that the first decision is to establish a priority for work training. Options are Wages and Integration, Skill Development and Choice, and Visibility.

For office use only
Priority:

Activity Order Form

Leisure Domain

1-1 Exercise
1-2 Games/Crafts/Hobbies
1-3 Events
1-4 Media
1-5 Other

Items Ordered			
Category	Item Number	Activity Description	Comments

Choose some items from each category. It is good to have a balance between things to do alone and things to do with others. It is also good to choose some activities that are constantly available and some that follow a schedule.

For office use only	
Total Items	
Total Categories Sampled	

Personal Management Domain

2-1 Self
2-2 Food
2-3 Space and Belongings
2-4 Personal Business

Items Ordered			
Category	Item Number	Activity Description	Comments

Choose activities from all categories. Select items that are important for the household.

For office use only	
Total Items	
Total Categories Sampled	

Work Domain

3-1 Agriculture and Natural Resources
3-2 Distribution
3-3 Domestic and Building Services
3-4 Food Preparation and Services
3-5 Office and Business Services
3-6 Construction
3-7 Health Occupations
3-8 Manufacturing and Machine Operations
3-9 Miscellaneous Occupations

Items Ordered		
Job Cluster	Support or Training Format	Comments

Possible support or training formats include Individual job, Crew or Enclave. Comments should include hours, possible tasks and location. Note that the first decision is to establish **a priority for work training**. Options are Wages and Integration, Skill Development and Choice, and Visibility.

For office use only
Priority: